Tales of the Exam Room Volume 5: **Amusing Medical Stories**

ISBN: 978-1-954814-11-0 (Paperback)

ISBN: 978-1-954814-10-3 (EBook)

First Edition 2022.

Credits:

Book Cover and Formatting by: farhanshahid101

Obsidian Wolf Publishing

PO Box 1086 Salem, UT 84653

Contents

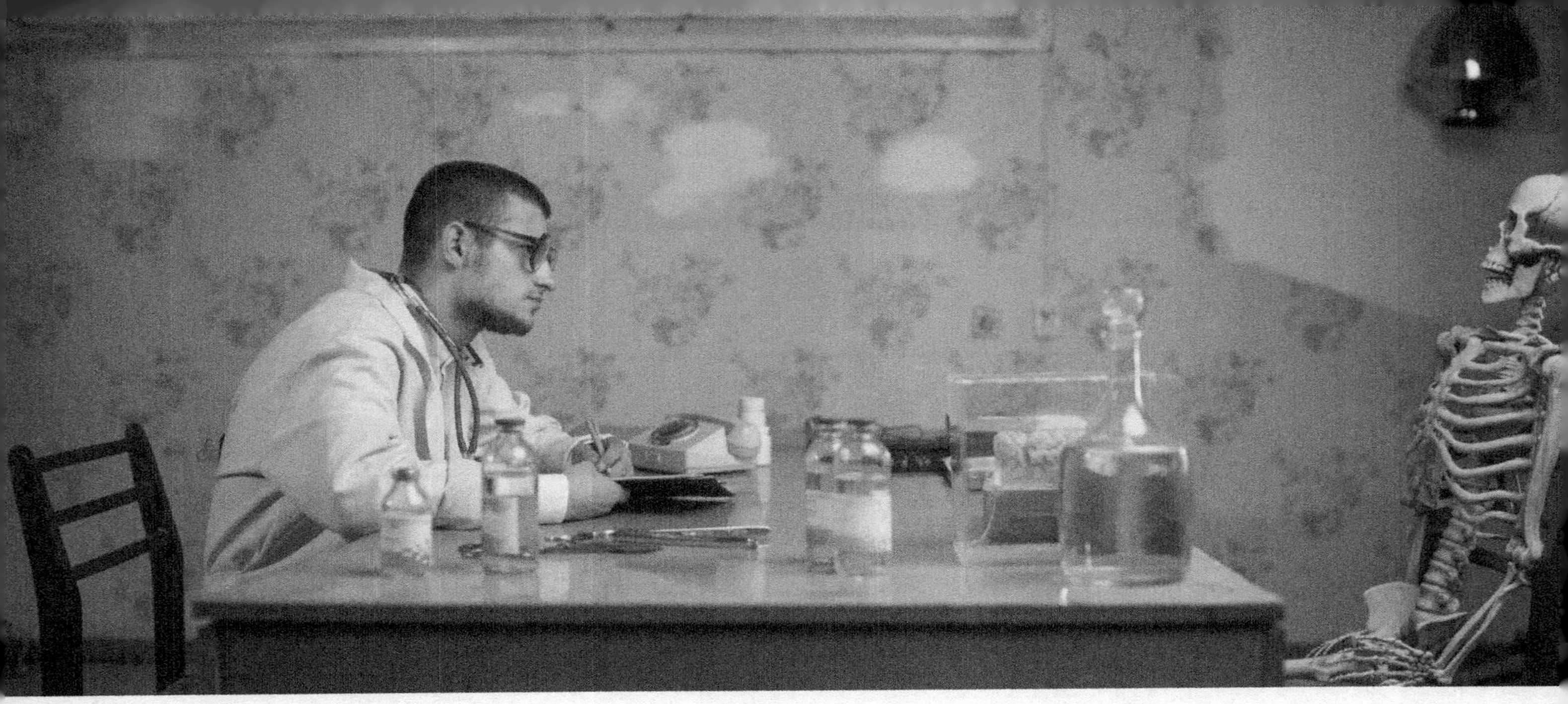

Introduction

Amusing Medical Stories: Tales of the Exam Room – Vol 5.

These tales are intended to be felt, enjoyed, and told repeatedly. There is so much to learn about patient encounters, decision-making disasters, and incredible actions of those involved during odd and life-saving situations.

Whether you come to this book having read the last four and enjoy our stories, or you are new to the wild world of crazy medical stories, we hope that you will enjoy this volume. If this is your first time, please check out our other four volumes.

Regardless of why you are here, you are in the right place. This is our 5th volume of short stories, and we hope that you find these slightly more humorous than the others, at least collectively.

We have collected amusing medical stories from a variety of different places and medical circumstances. We have changed the names, locations, and often the situations to protect the privacy and to provide a slightly more entertainment value.

This book is intended to cause the reader to shake their heads or question whether a particular episode truly happened. Most people love sitting around the dinner table or a campfire listening to unforeseen stories. Please understand that we are not poking fun at any particular person, situation, group, or otherwise.

Additionally, it is important to understand that fear, confusion, and lack of understand ng may play a role in some of the decisions made in these stories. Don't rush to be judgmental. These accounts will bring about a greater clarity into the unbelievable circumstances that medical professionals and patients find themselves in.

Volume 5 looks at some of the naiveties of sexual explorations, the confusion of the mind, food disasters, unbelievable accidents, and a case of medical isolation to the extreme.

Remember that the art of medicine is seldom straightforward and common sense is not always common. Please Enjoy and Feel free to Join Us for additional medical stories at examroomtales.com

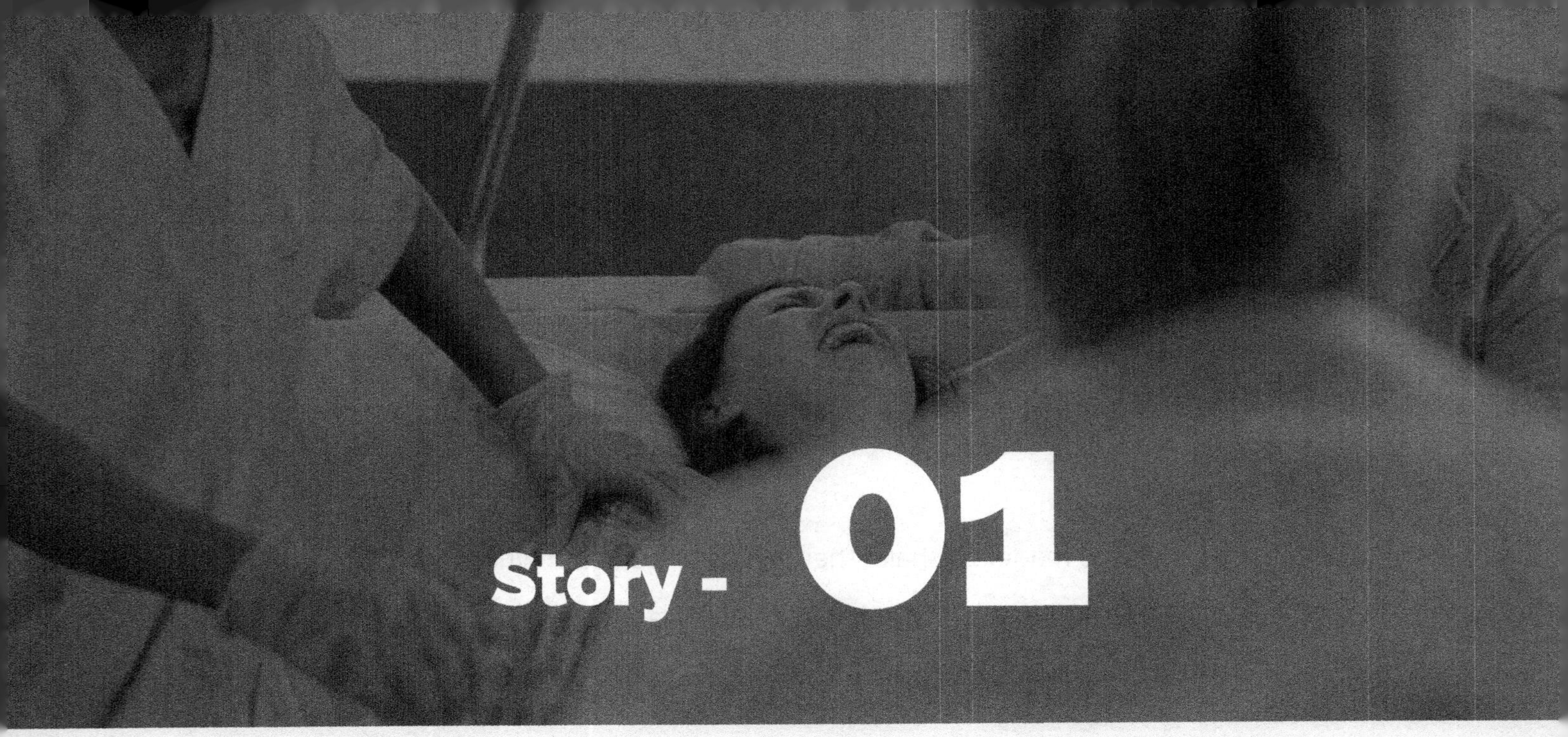

Emergency Risk of a Childbirth at the Prison

Pregnant women are sent to jails and prisons around the country, which can often become a complicated process. If they have less serious court cases or charges, they might remain in jail until a few weeks before they are supposed to deliver. Once the time comes, they will be released and allowed to deliver on their own terms and at their own cost. However, if their court cases are serious enough, they might be sentenced to prison, and in many cases, they will deliver while serving time for that case.

Either way, it is extremely rare for a patient to deliver at the jail or the prison. They are often brought to a local hospital for a few days for childbirth. A family member or adoption agency may get involved in determining where the child goes while the mother is incarcerated. In some cases, they will lose custody of the child. Each case is unique. After a few days, assuming there are no complications during childbirth, the inmate will be brought back to the prison. In just a handful of states, the baby will be allowed into the prison in a special area.

This next story comes from a prison where Darla Shumaker was sent for three years for her multiple crimes. She arrived at the jail reporting she was several months along and was sent to prison a month later. She anticipated serving two years in prison.

Dave McMillian was the nurse that arrived for his shift on that fateful day. The first half of his evening shift was challenging but manageable as he gathered supplies, passed medications, checked on patients, and took care of some medical issues in the women's unit. He was working an overnight shift. Sometimes things went smoothly, and sometimes they didn't. In this particular prison, the women's unit was a significant distance away from the men's unit. Dave had been busy going to different buildings during the first few hours.

Darla arrived at the prison and didn't mention her pregnancy until a few months after she arrived. However, she started having severe contractions just after three am. Darla started screaming and hollering, and her entire section was woken up. She lived in a dorm setting, and there were another seven girls in the same area. Soon, the girls had her comfortable, placed blankets around her, and rubbed her hands and feet. But the other girls were worried about her, and they contacted the closest officer.

Dave had just returned to his area from a different emergency when the phone started ringing.

Dave answered. "Hello."

"Is this a nurse?" asked an officer that Dave recognized.

"Hey Jacobs. Yea. It's me, Nurse Dave. What's going on?"

"It is Darla Shumaker. She has been on bed rest for pregnancy. She says that she got up to go to the bathroom, and everything was fine. Half an hour later, she's screaming and reporting her contractions are really close together."

"Okay."

"One of the other inmates came and said that Darla thinks her water broke."

"On my way." Dave grabbed a go-bag with essential supplies, including a blood pressure cuff, IV supplies, a delivery bag, and much more. As in every facility, the goal is for no female inmates to deliver at the prison. However, emergencies happen, and it's best to be prepared.

The nurse's office was a few minutes away from the unit, and Dave gathered the supplies, got into a cart, and drove to the unit. When he arrived, it was chaos. Five inmates and several officers were huddled around Darla. She was screaming and crying. Some of the women inmates were sitting near Darla. They had put a pillow and blanket on the inmate. Cool clothes were draped on her forehead. One of the older women was helping Darla to breathe calmly.

Dave rushed to the patient and placed a blood pressure cuff on her arm. He said, "Darla. I'm Nurse Dave, and we're going to help you. What happened?"

Through her tears, Darla said, "I don't know. I thought the pressure I was feeling meant I needed to use the bathroom. It didn't help, and then suddenly I felt sharp pains in my stomach. I've had two children before."

One of the other inmates added, "She told us about the pain, and she became so pale. She started holding her stomach, and that was when we noticed the puddle. I got up and told one of the other girls to get an officer."

"How long ago?"

"Ten minutes, maybe."

Turning back to Darla, Dave asked, "Then what happened?"

"I started feeling these strong contractions. I've had three other kids. These were far stronger than the Braxton-Hicks contractions I've been feeling for the last several months."

"How far along are you?"

Darla didn't answer this question. She began squeezing the hands of another inmate. Through gritted teeth, she said, "Another contraction." Darla's face contorted, and she began screaming. It was impossible to understand what she was saying.

Another officer added, "That is the fourth contraction since I've been here. All about five minutes apart."

"How far along are you?" Dave repeated.

"Eight months and some change," Darla hissed. Her face was bright red, and she was sweating.

Dave checked the blood pressure; it read 175/100. There was fluid on the floor and a wet spot between her legs and down one side.

"The baby wants to come," Darla screamed. "Should I push or not?"

Dave checked the belly. It was protruding out as if she could have a baby at any time. The abdomen was hard, and she screamed out in pain when he touched her stomach.

Into a radio, Dave said, "We need to call an ambulance to the women's prison. We have a possible emergency delivery."

The men and women around the section jumped into action. The ambulance was called. Chains were gathered, and a gurney was brought in by two other nurses. Dave began working on getting an IV started. Clothing and other supplies were collected by Darla's cellmate. The ambulance arrived quickly to the prison. Darla had another few contractions in the meantime. The entire time, two of the women inmates helped her breathe slowly and rubbed her forehead or her back.

"Don't push," Dave said. "Keep calm and keep breathing."

Darla was moved onto the gurney, and she had handcuffs placed on both arms. She was wheeled out of the section. Most of the women in the area came out and started clapping and yelling well wishes to Darla.

Dave and another nurse directed the gurney to the front of the building, where the ambulance was waiting. Once they arrived, the paramedics took over.

The first paramedic asked, "Give me the details."

Dave explained what was going on.

To Darla, the paramedic asked, "How far along?"

She replied quickly, "Thirty-eight weeks. My due date is in 12 days. It's a girl, my first. I've been in prison for five months. I've had four other children, all vaginal births. My BOGYN is Doctor Sheila Graves outside of prison. I have been seen weekly here in the prison. Last week I was dilated to a two."

They assessed her blood pressure, contractions, and IV placement. The paramedics thanked Dave and the other staff, put Darla into the back of the ambulance, and drove away.

Dave let out a long sigh of relief. He worked the remaining of his shift and went home the next morning.

He was scheduled to work later that night, and he was eager to get to work and find out what had happened with Darla. When he arrived, he noticed several balloons attached to his chair. Three pink balloons and one that read, "It's a girl!"

Dave was surprised at the welcoming gift. He had never known another nurse to get similar gifts. He found candy cigars lying on the top of his desk as he approached.

"Glad to see you, Dave," a voice said from the corner.

Dave glanced up to see his supervisor Dorian step into the room. "Congratulations on such a smooth departure."

"Did everything go okay with Darla?"

"As well as can be expected."

"Did something happen?"

"Nothing happened, except you got fooled."

"What are you talking about?"

"The ambulance arrived at the hospital, and they were ready for an emergency delivery. The funny thing is that she wasn't even pregnant."

"What?" Dave cried. "You've got to be kidding."

"Not at all." Dorian's smile grew.

Dave said, more to himself, "That's why her story changed a few different times." He had remembered her story changed a few different times on the estimated due date and the number of previous pregnancies. He had chalked it up to stress. "I'm an idiot."

"No! She faked out the paramedics and even a doctor. After an hour of her screaming and nothing happening, they decided to take another look. It took two additional ultrasounds to finally figure out that she wasn't pregnant. She was screaming and crying and sweating like crazy. The entire time she insisted that she was pregnant."

"I can't believe it. Was she faking the entire time, or was there something else going on?"

Dorian said, "She has convinced herself, the other inmates, and even some of the staff that she was pregnant. We had already done a few ultrasounds ourselves and three or four pregnancy tests over the last three months. The girl is completely convinced that she is pregnant. She told the hospital that she would sue them if her baby died."

"Unbelievable," Dave replied. "She had other inmates bringing her food and massaging her feet."

"From what the doctor of the unit said, she lost a baby a few years ago and now believes that she is pregnant all the time. It's likely that she urinated on herself. She has some serious PTSD and she's going to need some help."

"It's a girl!" shouted another nurse, and a few nurses stepped into the room.

The entire staff, especially Dave, would never forget this experience going forward. From now on, they double-checked that a patient being sent to the hospital was actually pregnant.

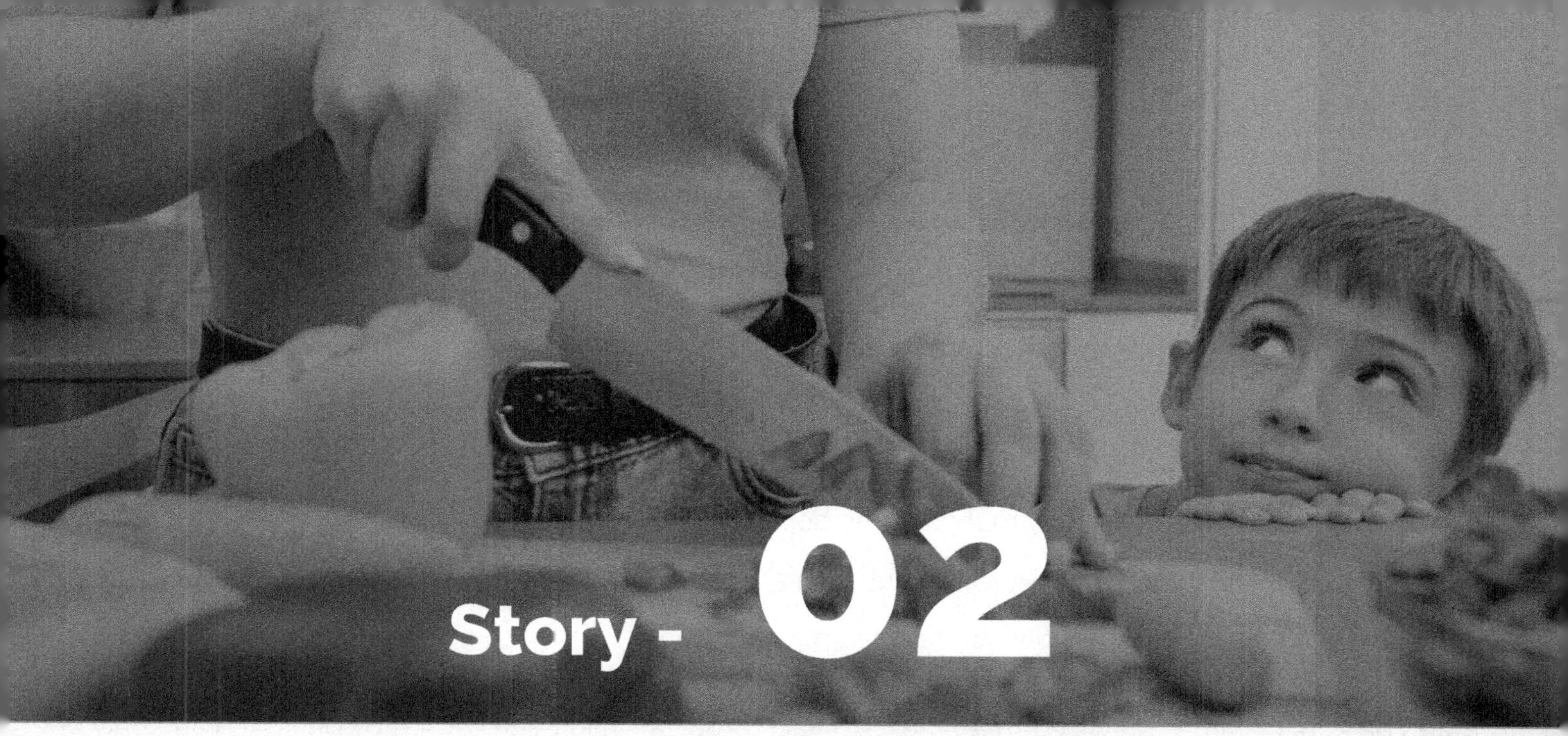

Story - 02

Boy with Orange Skin

Sam and Rebecca were amazing parents to their only son Brad. Over the years, they had noticed a substantial change in the nutrition choices of their child as he got older. It was easy to choose what he ate when he was young because he relied so much on his parents. As Brad began watching television and using his iPad, new advertisements for fast food, processed foods, and packaged foods were everywhere they looked. It didn't take long for him to decide against all vegetables.

Sam and Rebecca worked harder to point Brad in the right direction regarding healthy food options and potential consequences. It was extremely difficult to avoid junk food altogether, but they tried. All Brad wanted to eat at home or at school was sugary snacks, sugar cereal, and such. He would become angry if they tried anything different.

Soon, it was apparent that Brad loathed vegetables. He would throw a fit every time a vegetable was served for dinner or an after-school snack. They made the mistake of bribing Brad with video game time in order to eat some vegetables or a healthy snack. That soon backfired. Talking with other parents, it appeared that most of their friends struggled with the same problems.

When Brad was around thirteen, a few days after Halloween, he developed a severe stomach ache, and the parents first thought it was because of all the candy he was sneaking after Halloween. The next day, Brad was even worse, and he began vomiting uncontrollably. He had trouble standing because of all the pain. Brad was rushed to the hospital, where they found that his appendix was inflamed, infected, and about to burst. He was rushed into surgery and fortunately came out with a small scar and a short night spent in the hospital. Sam and Rebecca worried the entire time and came up with a plan.

Brad's parents became convinced that Brad's stomach problems had been caused by one thing and only one thing—his diet. They removed every sugary cereal, all his Halloween candy, any packaged chips, granola bars, and any other treat in the entire house. They replaced them with carrots, oranges, apples, and a ton more fruits and vegetables. At first, Brad didn't have a huge appetite, so it wasn't a big deal.

As time progressed, he became more and more hungry. He had no option but to pretend to love fruits and vegetables. At every meal, including breakfast, most of his food was vegetables. He was given salads and squash and yams. There was no way he could eat spinach, broccoli, or Brussels sprouts. To his genuine surprise, Brad learned that he liked most of the different types of fruit and some of the vegetables. He quickly realized that he loved carrots the most. But he still ate plenty of oranges, mangoes, and apricots.

Sugar cravings returned around the third or fourth week after surgery. He pleaded and pleaded with his parents to allow some sugary types of food. They were extremely hesitant. They felt that Brad's health was the best it had ever been, and they didn't want to rock the boat. Finally, they came to an agreement. If Brad ate around twenty carrots a day, they would allow him a granola bar or some applesauce.

Two weeks later, Rebecca's sister came to visit the family from out of town. Right away, she noticed that something was off with Brad.

After he had gone to bed, Cammie asked, "Rebecca? Have you noticed that your son's skin looks slightly yellow or maybe orange?"

"Not really," she said absentmindedly.

"Has he been sick?"

"Not since he had his appendix taken out. He's been so healthy and happy. It has been so good to watch. Sam and I feel so much better."

Cammie took out her phone and showed Rebecca some of the images. She found some pictures from before Brad had surgery and afterward. It didn't take long for Rebecca to notice the subtle difference in his skin color as well. She was surprised. She didn't know what to make of it, but her son's skin looked orange. She asked, "Could it be from his appendix surgery?"

"I'm not sure," Cammie replied. "Can you get an appointment with your doctor?"

"That's probably a good idea."

Rebecca telephoned their pediatrician the following day and was able to schedule an appointment for later that afternoon. Dr. Fineleson noticed the slight change in the color of Brad's skin the moment he walked into the room. He quickly started an exam and thought the color of the white area of his eyes was affected as well. Once he finished, he said, "He looks healthy, and everything else is just fine. I don't want to worry you, but we need to do some blood work."

Her sister Cammie had come along for the doctor's visit, and they shared a glance.

"What would you be looking for?" asked Rebecca

"Well," Dr. Fineleson replied. "Not sure exactly. There are conditions like jaundice, kidney problems, diabetes, and thyroid conditions that can cause skin color changes. It doesn't seem like those are likely, but it would be good to be thorough."

The blood work was done that day, and Rebecca, Cammie, and Brad were sent home to wait for the results. A few days later, they were called back into the pediatrician's office. Dr. Fineleson met them and said, "Good news. Most of the blood work came back normal. There are no kidney issues, diabetes, or other problems. There's nothing serious going on."

"So, what's going on? Do you know why my son's skin is orange?"

"I believe so."

"Well?" asked Rebecca.

"Too much of a good thing," replied Dr. Fineleson.

"What's that supposed to mean?" asked Rebecca.

"There was a large amount of beta-carotene levels in the blood. In other words, this means that Brad is getting too many vegetables."

Rebecca shook her head. "How's that possible?"

"How many carrots, oranges, and other vegetables is he eating?"

"A lot," replied Brad quickly.

Rebecca held up both hands and began explaining how she had heard that his poor diet might have caused his appendix surgery. Rebecca and Brad's father had agreed to cut out processed foods along with sugary foods and anything else unhealthy.

Dr. Fineleson nodded and listened. "That makes sense," he said at last. "Brad had a condition called Carotenemia. I've never seen it before, but a colleague of mine has. It happens when a patient consumes way too many carotene-rich foods such as carrots, oranges, and more. The liver gets a little overwhelmed, and your skin can turn orange or yellow."

"Is it dangerous?" asked Rebecca.

"Not at all. Though it probably isn't advised either. Eating this many carrots and other vegetables to cause this type of skin reaction isn't as healthy as you might think. Equally important is the understanding that sweets likely didn't cause his appendicitis either. Balance is the key."

"How do we stop it?"

"Nothing impossible. Just make sure that Brad eats only eat a few vegetables a day. You don't need to go overboard."

"Can I have sugar cereal and snacks?"

"That's up to your mom," Dr. Fineleson replied. "I wouldn't go overboard on sugary snacks either. Drink plenty of water, get some exercise, a normal amount of sleep, and remember to balance things out."

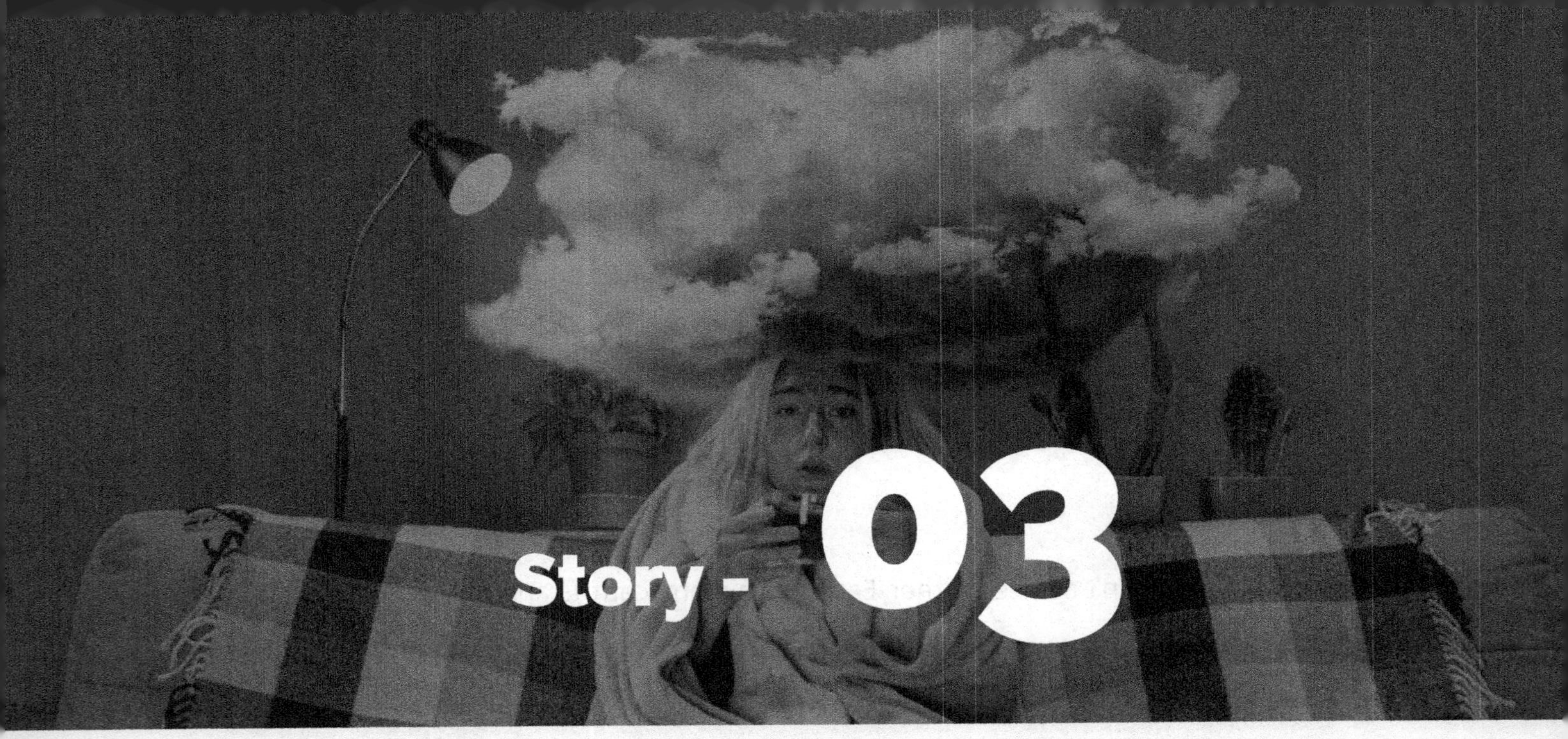

A Cough that Turned into a Circus

One of the worst medical days of my career was several years ago while I worked in a remote same-day medical clinic. We had a small number of scheduled appointments, and most of our patients just showed up and were seen in the order they arrived. It was the doctor, the receptionist and me. When I say remote, I mean remote.

Our clinic was open Monday through Friday, but if there was a real emergency, ultrasound, or X-ray, the patients often had two choices. They could drive an hour to the nearest hospital or wait until the tech came out for the following visit. X-rays would come out twice a week, and ultrasounds once a week. It was usually Thursdays for our ultrasounds, which included our pregnant patients and other necessary evaluation processes. I usually called these patients Wednesday night to remind them to drink water or arrive at the clinic with a full bladder. X-rays were Mondays and Fridays, and they usually didn't have special instructions.

Susan Ray came to the clinic on a Tuesday and was asked by the receptionist what her complaint was. Susan reported that it was a cough with fever and chills. Indeed, it was nearing flu season, and Susan wasn't the only person in our clinic that week with this complaint. The receptionist gave her paperwork to fill out and told her to take a seat until she was called into the back. Our receptionist, Betty, is incredible. She will watch each patient who comes through the doors while they are waiting, and she will write down a few notes on what she sees.

Susan filled out the appropriate paperwork and provided an insurance card. Susan Ray was reasonably familiar with how things worked, and she had been seen in the clinic several times over the last few years. This was the first time she had been in the clinic this year. She had Diabetes, Hypertension, and here and there problems with arthritis and heartburn.

Susan probably coughed four or five times in the twenty minutes she waited to be brought back to a room. There were eight people in the waiting room when she arrived. We were normally efficient and could place three people in the exam rooms at a time. On this Tuesday, we did a great job. Our waiting room is relatively small, and people need to sit close by each other. Not once, while Susan was coughing, did she cover her mouth. A few other patients wanted to move, but they had no place to go. Otherwise, Susan was very talkative to the other guests in the waiting room. They shared a few stories and talked about why they were there.

I brought Susan back to her room. Her weight was down five pounds from last year, and her blood pressure was well controlled. She told me that she had been eating better and exercising. Once in the room, I started asking her about recent problems, new issues, and current symptoms related to her cough. She had no history of asthma or other breathing issues. She had hot and cold flashes. She told me that these symptoms happened because of the dry air this time of year and had been going on for two weeks. Her farm had a lot of dust, and she had been outside as much as possible.

"Anything else?" I asked.

"No, darling. That's it."

I nodded and left to get the doctor.

Doctor Valentine entered the room. He started with some small talk and asked how Susan Ray's family was. Susan was happy and told a few funny stories. Her kids had left the house, but one was close by, and they had Sunday dinner weekly. The other three kids had moved to the city.

Doctor Valentine continued, "Well, Susan. Nurse Jamie tells me that you aren't feeling well."

"I have this terrible cough."

"How often do you feel that you cough? A few times during the day? Is it worse at night?"

"Oh, yes. It has been terrible. It is substantially worse during the day, but it is still a problem at night. It wakes me up sometimes. I feel like I am soaking wet all the time. The nurse said that I had lost a ton of weight. I barely have an appetite and feel so weak and tired all the time."

Doctor Valentine glanced at me momentarily. He asked, "How long has this been going on?"

"Five or six weeks," replied Susan.

"What do you think could be causing this?"

"I don't know, doctor. But I am really sick. My kids are worried. They almost forced me to go into town to get tested."

There was a knock at the door, and I went to open it. Betty, our receptionist, stood there, and she whispered, "We have a problem in the waiting room. Several of the patients are refusing to leave."

I told Doctor Valentine that I would be back.

Stepping out of the door, I heard Susan Ray say something about being on a cruise ship a month ago, and I shook my head as I closed the door. She had never said anything about a cruise or most of her symptoms. When I walked into the waiting room, there was a flurry of commotion.

Several patients were upset. I asked what was going on, and they told me that they were distraught because they had just had an exposure to tuberculosis. I was confused and it tock a moment for my mind to catch up to what they were saying. I asked everyone to sit down, and I picked one patient, Jimmy Sanders, to give me an explanation.

"What's going on Jimmy?"

He said, "I was sitting two people away from that woman, Susan Ray. She started coughing on all of us. You all saw it. She refused to cover her mouth and told us that it didn't matter because she had tuberculosis and was about to die anyway."

"Tuberculosis?" I asked. "Are you sure?"

"That's what she said."

Other patients confirmed Jimmy's story. They were seriously freaked out.

I said, "Let me go talk to Doctor Valentine, and I'll tell you what needs to happen."

"Don't take forever. If I need to go to the hospital, we will need to take off before it gets too late," replied Jimmy.

I quickly hurried off and knocked on the door. I opened it a crack and asked for Doctor Valentine to step out of the room.

"What is it nurse Jaime?"

"Apparently, Susan Ray told everyone in the waiting room that she has tuberculosis and is going to die. They're agitated and want to know what they should do."

"Susan Ray said this to them?"

"That's what they're saying." I added, "She told me that her cough was from the dry air from her farm."

Doctor Valentine appeared puzzled. "She just told me that she has a family history of Asthma."

"Something is off about her," I said.

Together we went back into the room. Doctor Valentine said, "Have you been telling people in the lobby that you have tuberculosis?"

"I might have mentioned it," Susan replied.

"Do you know what TB is?" asked Doctor Valentine.

"A condition caused by a bacteria called Mycobacterium tuberculosis, and the bacteria attacks your lungs. It is spread through the air when someone coughs, sneezes, or talks."

"Okay," said Doctor Valentine. "How do you know that you have TB?"

"Um," replied Susan. "I got an X-ray while I was on the cruise ship."

I asked, "Why didn't you mention to me that you had been on a cruise ship?

Doctor Valentine said, "If you had been diagnosed on a cruise ship, you likely would have been quarantined."

I added, "You kept telling me that your cough was from the dust at your farm."

"Coughs can be caused by multiple things Nurse Jaime."

Doctor Valentine said, "I did an exam, and you expressed to me about a possible family history of asthma."

"Another potential cause."

"Tuberculosis can be identified by a blood test and a Chest X-ray. We will order both to find out what is happening. X-ray will be here in a few days, and we can send out the blood work today."

"My kids are concerned that I am going to die."

"We will make sure that we find out what is really going on."

The other patients were placed on a list to be notified, and they were told that additional testing was needed. For now, they shouldn't worry but they should stay home until they get the results.

The next day, when I showed up at the clinic, it was closed. The county's health department had been notified about a possible exposure to TB. Doctor Valentine, myself, and Betty were unable to work because of the exposure, and the clinic was shut down.

In the end, Susan Ray did not have tuberculosis. Testing was done immediately for her at the local hospital. It still took three days to get cleared to reopen. I was poked and prodded myself. I had to get an X-ray and give some blood samples. It was a terrible experience. Every night I played the "What if" game. I couldn't help myself.

On Friday, Susan arrived early at the clinic to apologize. She said, "I was so worried about my cough, and my kids wouldn't listen to what I was saying. I went on a cruise a year ago and did have some issues with coughing. But I guess it really isn't that bad."

I asked, "What about tuberculosis."

"My son searched on the internet and came over this last Sunday. He was convinced that I had tuberculosis and he convinced me that I did as well. I didn't know about the testing and what TB really was. I am so sorry."

"No problem," Doctor Valentine said. "My staff and I needed a little vacation, hazmat suits, plenty of blood tests, and it was good to have a getaway. Now, we're ready to get back to work."

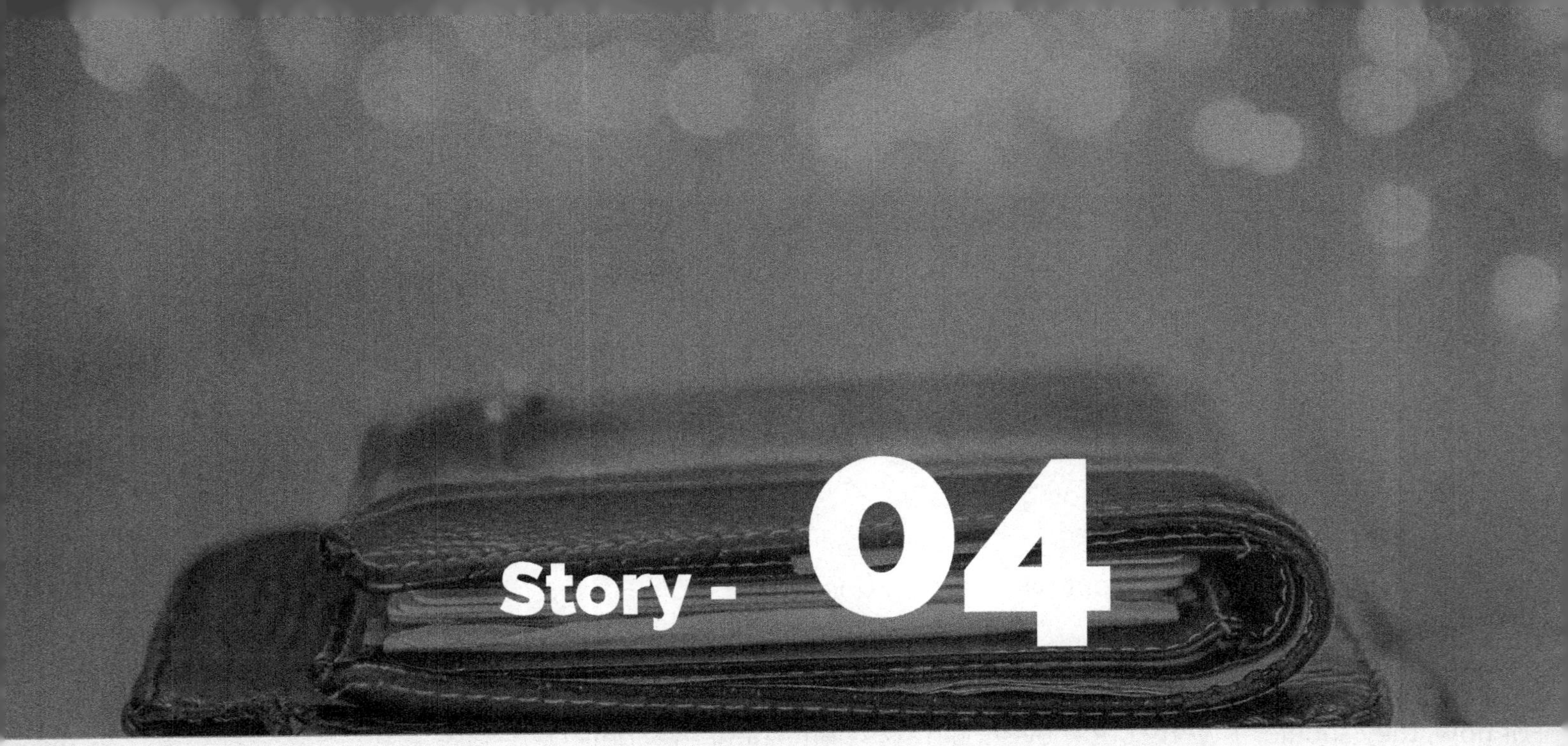

Story - 04

You Keep That in Your Wallet?

A male patient came into our clinic and was extremely upset, wanting to see one of our medical staff immediately. He didn't have an appointment, but he had come with two girls who waited outside in the waiting room. At the check-in, he was nearly hysterical. He was added to the clinic list with one of our providers. I was the nurse assigned to his room and had heard him screaming for a full five minutes before he was calm enough to explain why he was there. Once inside his room, I tried listening to his complaints to better understand what he was going through.

During the conversation, he jumped from one issue to another and wasn't making much sense. He was upset about his girlfriends finding out about each other, other random girls, a call from the health department, and a possible infection. He spoke about filing a lawsuit against the condom makers, the television station, and all his doctors. He insisted that these things shouldn't have happened to him. It took me a good twenty minutes to calm him down.

He stayed quiet enough for me to check his vitals. They were normal. Suddenly, he began to hyperventilate and tried explaining things again. Five minutes later, he was ready to start at the beginning. As he talked and explained his situation, he paced back and forth in the small room. He was distraught because his two girlfriends hadn't known about each other until he was forced to talk with both of them last night. He was twenty-two and felt the burden of going to school, working part-time, and trying to make ends meet. I asked him questions about his health, medications, and any history of medical problems in his family. He finally calmed down and was willing to answer the questions and explain precisely why he was in our clinic.

He said, "My name is Jared Collins, and I need to get fixed."

"Jared," I said. "What sort of phone call did you get from the health department?"

"It was from a nurse, and she said that I was a sexual partner of someone who recently tested positive for an STD."

"Did she say what kind of STD?"

"What did you say your name was?" he asked.

"Nurse Irene."

"Okay, Nurse Irene," said Jared. "The health department said it was a disease that is passed sexually, but it is treatable."

I replied, "Typically, that could mean Chlamydia or Gonorrhea."

Jared answered, "Those both could be possibilities. I really can't remember exactly what she called them."

"We can do a test and check."

Jared interrupted. "They said that I could just get a treatment, and that would fix everything."

"Most STDs can be treated with an antibiotic or two depending on the cause."

"Fine," said Jared. His voice became firm when he asked, "Nurse Irene, aren't STDs preventable?"

"Yes. Prevention means something you do before you get the STD, such as birth control or condoms."

"I don't think that any of my girlfriends use birth control by I use a condom."

"Was the call from the health department about your girlfriends?"

"No. It was about a girl that I met at a campus party."

"Did you use a condom with her?"

"Oh, yes. I always do. That's why I want to sue the condom makers. There's no way that I could have an STD."

"Well," I explained. "That's not what the health department is saying. They will contact all those who have a potential sexual exposure, and it seems like you were on the list."

"What are my risks if I did use a condom?"

"If you used it correctly, the risks are really low. Let me go talk with the doctor and see what he wants to do." I left the room and found Doctor Gerard. When I came back, I explained, "The doctor would like to test you just to make sure."

"If he thinks so," replied Jared. "Can my two girlfriends be checked as well?"

"We would recommend that they get tested as well."

"They're here. In the waiting room."

"Okay," I said. "Why are they here?"

"They want to be part of the lawsuit against the condom makers."

I shook my head. "We'll test them as well."

A few days later, all three individuals returned to the clinic for their results. They were each placed in a separate room and explained the results. All three were beyond shocked. They each ended up testing positive for an STD. They demanded to be brought to the same room for further explanation. I went in to talk with them, and Jared was livid and upset. All he wanted to do was blame the condom makers. He ranted and raved about things going wrong even when you tried to do the right thing. The two girls had just recently met each other and assured me that their only sexual partner was Jared.

After a lengthy conversation about risk factors and transmission issues, Jared admitted that he had a few different sexual partners but that these two girlfriends were his only loves. He assured me that he used a condom in all cases, and he couldn't imagine how they could've possibly gotten an STD.

"Look," I said. "The important part is that we need to treat all of you. It'll take a shot and some oral medications, and you can be treated."

"When can we have sex again?" asked Jared.

"Not for a week or so," I replied.

"This is not fair," cried Jared again.

I glanced over at one of the girls and noticed that she seemed different. She had a glow about her. A thought suddenly came into my mind. I replied, "Before we start treatment, I would like to talk to each of you individually and potentially get some more testing."

"Why," asked Jared.

"Just to make sure that we get everything taken care of today."

I again spoke to the doctor, and he agreed to allow a pregnancy test on the two girls. After some gentle nudging, they both consented to the testing. The girl with the glow turned out to be pregnant while the other girl wasn't. I gave the information to the girl, and she stormed into Jared's room and questioned him.

Jared responded, "That's impossible. The condom is clearly at fault. It didn't protect anyone from getting an STD, and now this. This is condom malpractice."

Both girls were emotional, confused, and uncomfortable. The situation went from bad to worse right before my eyes.

I asked, "Are you using a condom every time you have sex?"

"I wear it each time," he replied with a fierce look on his face. "If you want, you can look at it?"

"What do you mean?" I asked.

"I bring the condom with me wherever I go."

I laughed. "You mean that you bring condoms, and you keep one in your wallet or somewhere else."

"No. I use the same one, and I wash it out every time. I even use soap."

"No way," I cried.

Pulling out his wallet, he removed a small plastic bag and put it on the exam table. I nearly lost it.

I screamed, "One condom is intended to be used for one time, and then you throw it away. You don't clean and reuse condoms."

"Are you sure?" He glanced at the girls. "That's not what my brother told me."

"I'm a hundred percent positive. You probably got a hole in it or something. It's useless."

"Huh," said Jared. "Why didn't you tell me that in the first place? It is obvious that condom makers need to take a little more responsibility in explaining how to use them. A package insert would be nice, wouldn't it?".

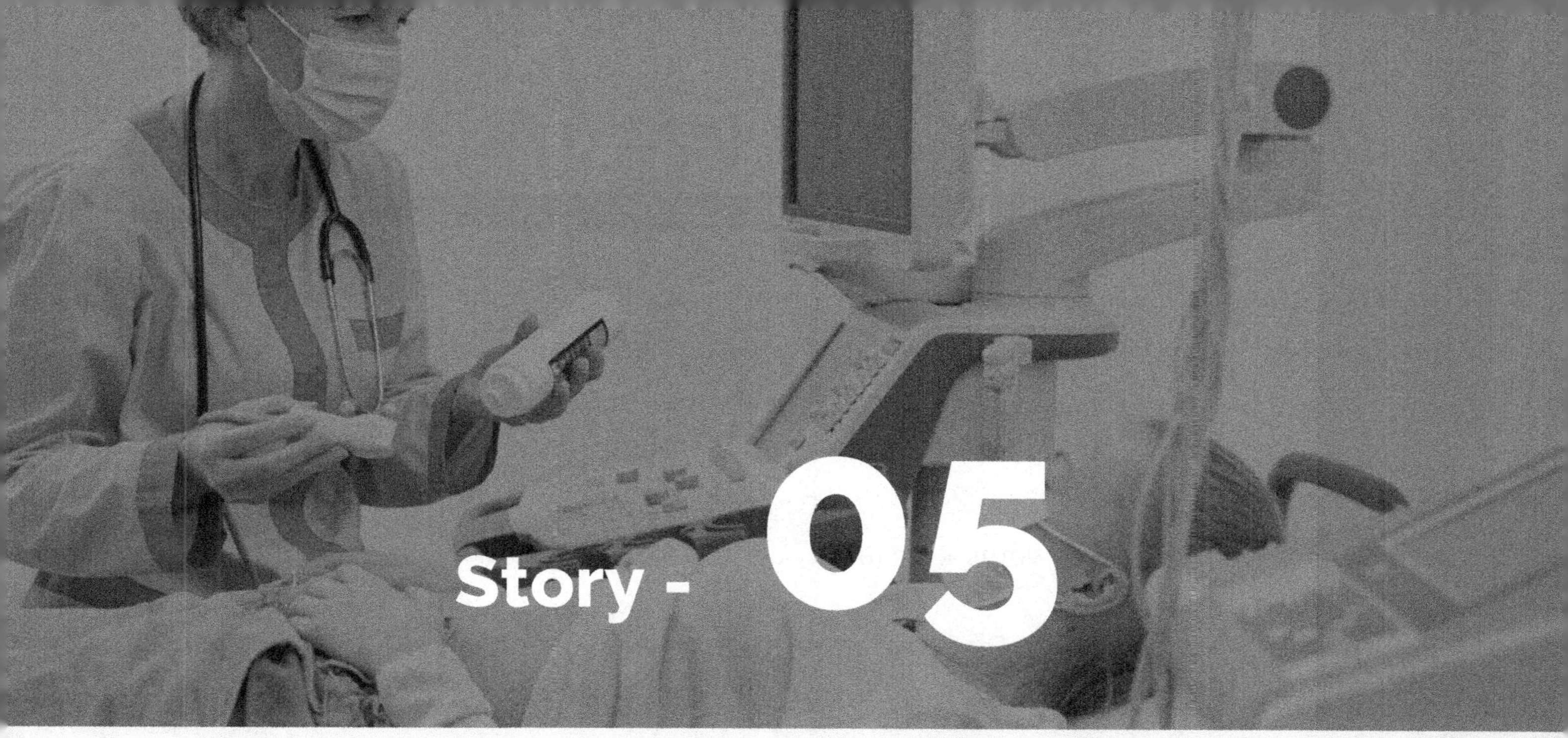

Secrets in a Hidden Special Place

An individual brought into the county jail following an arrest for drugs, theft, and assault became one of the weirdest situations I've seen in my twenty-two year career. The police had caught her selling and using drugs, and when she spotted them, she ran in hopes of finding a way to escape. The officers followed and found her in an abandoned building, hiding in one of the rooms. The officers tried talking with her, but she refused to answer or cuff up. Stepping forward to arrest her, she lashed out, screaming and flailing her arms. She hit the officers a few times in the process.

Upon arrival at the jail, she refused to get out of the car and tried grabbing ahold of anything she could. This isn't completely unusual. She was talking gibberish, and drool was coming out of her mouth. It was as if she had lost her mind. She kept mumbling and talking to someone who wasn't there. She picked at her skin hard. Once inside, she adamantly refused to see a nurse, be fingerprinted, have her picture taken, and pretty much everything else. She was well known to the jail, and this type of behavior for her was usual. She was challenging and combative until she came off of her drugs and sobered up.

Nurse Phillip approached the patient in her cell and tried talking with her. "Ms. Bly. We need to get a urine sample to check if you're pregnant and to see if there are any other issues."

"Screw you and your mom and the president of the United freaking States," shouted Bambi Bly. "I'm not doing anything you ask." This time, her words were mostly understandable, but she slurred them.

"You just left jail a few weeks ago. Do you remember me helping you when you went through withdrawals the last time? I gave you something to drink and your medications."

"You're the devil's spawn of underwater mermaids, and I've never seen you before."

"Well. I'll come back and check on you again in half an hour. Maybe you'll remember me by then."

Bambi did not remember the nurse and spent the next several hours in a mania state followed by twelve hours of deep sleep. She was monitored closely by jail and medical staff. When she woke up the following day, she was somewhat better. She was still paranoid and confused and certainly did not want to be in jail. She was provided some fluids to drink and some Jell-o to eat. After keeping this down, nurse Phillip returned to talk with Bambi.

"Hello, Ms. Bly. How are you feeling today?"

"Die you coward!"

"We need to get your nursing assessment done."

"Leave me alone."

"I can once we make sure that we get your medications reordered and make sure there aren't other problems."

"Fine."

With the help of an officer, the patient was brought to a separate office for a nursing assessment. The officer remained in the room the entire time. At one point, Bambi said, "I swallowed a whole bunch of meth, and I stuck a pipe in my hidden area. Are you going to get that out?"

Nurse Phillip replied, "We can order an X-ray to see what you have placed in there. Unless you want to take it out yourself."

"I can do that."

The patient was moved to a different room, and she removed two balloons of heroin and small pieces of tinfoil items and other things. She said, "I guess the meth pipe was the last time I was here."

Bambi finished her medical screening and was brought to the infirmary for close monitoring. She was placed in a cell where she could be closely monitored by the nurses and other staff. She was given medications, fluids, and other things to help with her withdrawals. The nurses monitored her several times, and her behavior, confusion, and withdrawals improved gradually over time. She refused the X-ray that was ordered.

About five days after arriving, the doctor was passing by her cell, and Bambi Bly called her over. The doctor was performing her rounds, and she had already spoken a few times to Ms. Bly over the last few days.

"Doctor," Bambi said. "Please help me. I have a huge problem, and you are the only one who can help me."

"What kind of problem?" asked Dr. Duncan.

"I have something stuck in my vagina."

"I heard that you had brought in some drugs and such when you were first searched."

"No. This is something else. Can I be seen in the clinic?"

"Why did you refuse your X-ray when they were looking for the meth pipe?"

"It's not a meth pipe," she said flatly.

Ms. Bly was brought down to the exam room. A female officer - Fuller and nurse Otterson were present. Dr. Duncan said, "Ms. Bly. What is going on today?"

"I'm freaking out that I lost something. Maybe it fell into the toilet while I wasn't looking."

Dr. Duncan asked, "What would you have lost?"

"A piece of jewelry that is near and dear to my heart."

"As you know, when you are brought into jail, all of your property was placed in a bag for you to retrieve once you leave jail. Maybe this piece of jewelry is in your property and not lost."

"I know. But the nurses were kind enough to go looking in my property, and they didn't find the necklace."

"Could the necklace be somewhere else? Maybe in your car or at your home."

"I don't think so."

"You were disoriented when you arrived at the jail. Maybe you could call someone and have them search for the necklace."

"I have no one that could help me. The last thing I remember was stuffing it in my vagina for safekeeping."

Dr. Duncan glanced at the officer and the nurse. She asked. "Was an officer with Ms. Bly when she pulled out the other times?"

"Yes," replied officer Fuller. "It was someone that I work with. She pulled out some balloons of meth and a few more things. I don't think a necklace was removed."

"It has to be up there. Maybe it moved around or fell out."

After another moment of thought, Dr. Duncan said, "I can order you another X-ray. The soonest it can be done is tomorrow. The necklace will have metal, and if it happens to be there, we will find out."

"Thank you so much," replied Bambi.

"Why is this necklace so important to you."

"It's a family heirloom."

Nurse Otterson asked, "Is it from your grandmother or something? Is it old and valuable?"

"Oh no. I was adopted and in foster care for years and years. This is an heirloom from my family. It is something I bought after my boyfriend overdosed and died. We were going to get married."

"He was your fiancé?" asked Dr. Duncan, feeling slightly confused.

"I had seen him around on the streets. I think I even did drugs with him a few times in an abandoned building before I really connected with him. One time, we nearly were caught by the cops, and we hid together in a field for like hours. We ended up falling in love with each other right there, and we hung out every day for like three weeks. He didn't have anyone else either, and he told me that I made him feel special. I miss him so much. The heirloom helps me think of him whenever I am about to do drugs. It reminds me of what we could have had. He told me that he wanted to marry me when he got sober."

"That's cute...in a weird sort of way," replied Dr. Duncan.

"I know."

"What is the necklace?"

"It has a chain and two sets of metal teeth. They are the coolest thing ever."

"Okay," replied nurse Otterson. "What kind of heirloom is this?"

"Well," Bambi said, and her voice dropped. "I was able to get some blood from my boyfriend, and his sister gave me some of his ashes. Each tooth opens," and she used her hands to show that she was unscrewing a lid, "...and you can put a little bit into each side. You close it tight, and I have some of my boyfriend with me all at all times. I keep the necklace close to my heart or in my private place. It makes me feel calm and better about life. If it is missing, I'm going to die."

"Thanks for sharing," replied Dr. Duncan, feeling slightly nauseous. "We will get that X-ray ordered right away and figure out what happened to your necklace."

The following day, the X-ray was scheduled and done. Turned out, the chain and the two metal pieces, like teeth, were clearly visible. Dr. Duncan and the entire staff were amazed and horrified at the findings. The metal had wrapped itself around like a ball.

Dr. Duncan called Ms. Bly back in and told her of the results.

"Oh. Thank you. Thank you. Thank you." Bambi was so relieved, but she tried and tried and could not remove it herself.

Dr. Duncan said, "That means that I will have to go in and remove it. Are you okay with that?"

"As long as you don't break it."

"I won't."

Dr. Duncan performed an exam and was able to get the necklace removed with minimal issues. There was some slight bleeding of the skin afterward as it had clamped onto some of the skin.

Bambi was eternally grateful to know that she hadn't lost her necklace. She became quite a bit more upset when she learned that she could not keep the necklace with her during her stay in jail. She held onto it for a long time. Finally, it was taken to her property with her other items, and it would be waiting for her when she was released.

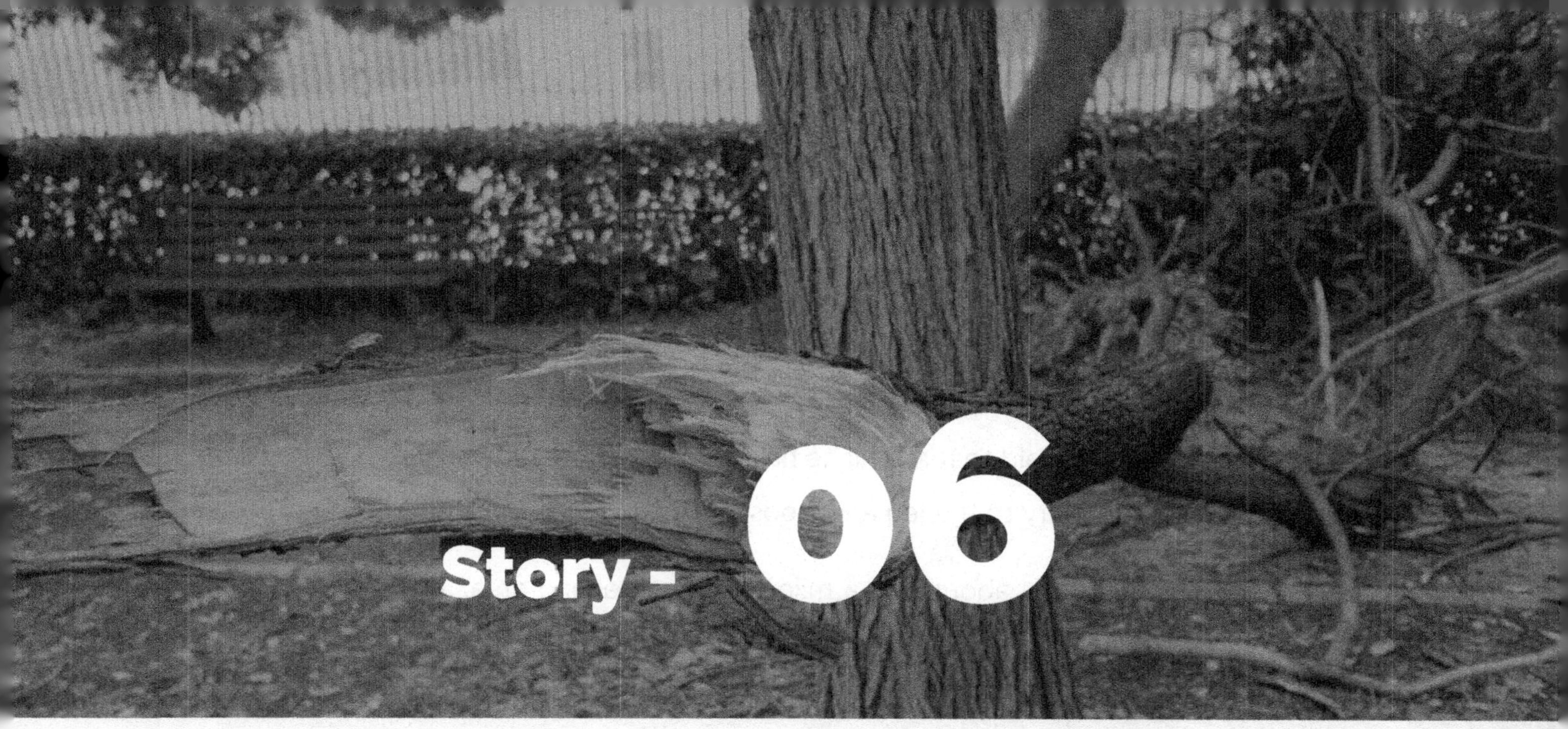

Story - 06

Is it an ATV Accident or a Possible Amputee?

A paramedic was finishing lunch at a local restaurant with his partner and a local high school student taking an emergency medicine high school class and getting some experience with a ride-along. They had just paid for their food when the call came in that there was an accident with a possible amputee scenario on one of the local trails near the National Park. It was far too windy to send in a Flight for Life helicopter. Their ambulance was the closest medical transport vehicle to the injury.

The drive up the canyon was scheduled to take more than twenty minutes, and they went as fast as they could. They had received very little additional information. A hiker had run down the mountain to get into cell service, and he reported an accident or a fall, though he didn't see the injured directly. They considered getting search and rescue involved, but apparently, the location was close to the trail, and the man's location was known to the group. The ambulance was required because the guy was in bad shape, and he needed to get to the hospital.

When the ambulance arrived, they found one man had been sent down the hill. He didn't have any updates. As they got things ready, He described hearing a whine of an engine, a crash, and a lot of screaming. Other people were there, and he was told to run until he had cellphone coverage and call the authorities. Someone had shouted about a severe injury to the leg and a possible need for an amputation.

The location of the accident was about half a mile from the parking area, and they would need to travel through some rugged terrain. They wouldn't be able to transport their gurney and decided to carry a plastic backboard, a medical bag, and some straps to get the patient stabilized.

It took more than fifteen minutes to get to the location. The area was in a pine forest with several different trails. This area appeared to be where motorcycles and ATVs often came for fun. Hikers and campers were also prevalent in this area. Some steep trails led to waterfalls further up the mountain.

"Over here," cried one of the guys when they came into view.

Derrick, the lead paramedic, was instructed to a cliff area to the right. Danvers was his partner, and Lincoln was the high school student.

They crossed off the trail and cut through some of the trees. At one point, they hit a ridge, and the path sloped down until it reached a substantial drop of ten feet. It was a hard climb to the bottom.

"I'm fine. What the hell is going on?"

"Jessie," a man shouted. "You're seriously injured. You knocked yourself out. The ambulance is here to help."

"I don't need any damn help."

For the first time, Derrick saw the accident scene. An ATV was off to the right side, face down. Steam came up from the engine.

"Help me get up," cried Jessie.

"Not until you're cleared by medical. They are almost here. I see them."

"Damn it. Tell them to hurry up."

Derrick shouted, "Jessie. We're the paramedics, and we're almost to you. Stay calm, and we can help you." To Danvers, he said, "You go find out what happened. Be quick about it." To Lincoln, he said, "Where do you want to go?"

Lincoln said, "With you. I want to see the injury." The excitement in the student's voice made Derrick smile.

Derrick took the backboard, and Lincoln was handed the straps. Derrick already had an emergency bag with supplies, gauze, a neck brace, and more. To get to Jessie and the three men around him took some maneuvering. They crossed back and forth and finally reached the lower area. Jessie was lying face down on the ground. Derrick could see that a leg and arm were broken even from here. He had a single blanket laid over his back.

Derrick said, "The guy you sent down the hill reported a possible amputee problem."

"No," shouted one of the men. It was the same guy who had been talking to Jessie earlier. "He had an ATV accident. He was going, and his wheel bent low, and his weight shifted, and he rolled down the hill. I'm pretty sure the ATV landed on him once."

"Who are you?"

"Tom Smiley."

"Okay, Tom. You're the voice for the group. I want to hear things from you only for the first few minutes. Later, if someone else has something to add, they can."

"Okay."

"How long was Jessie unconscious?"

"Thirty minutes or so. At first, he was just lying there. His leg looked bent wrong, and we were afraid to move him. We weren't sure what else we should do."

"Did you try to move him?"

"No."

"When he woke up, did he know where he was?"

"Mostly."

Jessie replied, "I asked what the hell happened."

His friends laughed.

Derrick asked Jessie, "Does your neck hurt? Can you feel your legs?"

"I can feel everything. I'm fine."

"Well," replied Derrick. "That's not exactly true. I'm down looking at your leg, and your bone is sticking through your skin. Most people would be screaming in pain."

Derrick turned to ask Lincoln to help, but Lincoln was on the ground, unconscious. He was pale but breathing. Derrick yelled, "Danvers. Over here! The high school student is out."

Danvers arrived and began checking Jessie's neck, who reported some pain but could feel everything in his legs and feet and could move his hands. Danvers pulled out a C-collar and began placing it on his neck.

Jessie argued, "See. I'm fine. Nothing is wrong with me. Why am I laying on the ground like this?"

Derrick and Danvers shared a glance. Derrick answered, "You've been in an accident, Jessie. You have a broken bone and were knocked unconscious. We will need to get you onto a backboard and strap you down. You have a head injury and possibly some more damage."

"No way. Everything feels fine." The wind started howling around the group as leaves and dirt were blown everywhere.

"I'm looking at your leg. I can see your bone."

Tom said, "You just told him that. Why are you saying it again?"

"Screw you," shouted Jessie. "You never said anything to me. This is the first time the doctor has said something to me since I arrived at the hospital."

Tom glanced over, confused.

Derrick mouthed, pointing to his own head, "A head injury. He needs to calm down. Let us get him to the ambulance."

"Sorry, Jessie," Tom said. "Just trying to help."

"Why is there blood dripping from my forehead?"

Having finished getting the C-collar into place, Danvers moved to get a good look at Jessie's face. "Oh, yea. Large laceration on forehead. Lots of bleeding. There might be some other injuries that I can't see."

"Everything else seems stable. He has a broken wrist, but it isn't a compound fracture."

"What now?" asked Danvers.

"We need to stabilize his head and roll him over to the backboard." The storm coming intensified, and rain started falling.

Danvers said, "Your student is starting to wake up."

"Leave him," Derrick shouted. "He'll be fine."

They positioned the backboard on the ground next to Jessie. They had to move some leaves and some branches and brushed the ground to make it as even as possible. It was starting to get a little wet. This was going to be a difficult move to get him onto the board. Danvers protected the head and neck, and the three guys and Derrick positioned themselves correctly, ready to turn Jessie.

"On the count of three," Derrick shouted. "One...two...three."

Jessie started to move but began screaming loudly. Ouch. Ouch. My stomach. Something is being ripped out of my stomach."

"Stop," Derrick shouted, and he quickly moved to the opposite side and bent low to the ground.

His mouth gaped open. Somehow Jessie had landed directly onto a tree stump, and it had sunk deep into his chest cavity. The tree's diameter was but a few inches, but it was directly into his center. Derrick asked, "Anyone have a shovel or something?"

"We do," screamed someone from back on top. A minute later, a small hand shovel used to dig up the ground when using the restroom was brought forward.

Lincoln had recovered enough to come help keep the body positioned safely as Derrick began chopping and digging the tree. He was pale but steady.

It took several long minutes, but finally, Derrick was able to cut through the tree. Jessie was screaming the entire time. The adrenaline of the moment was wearing off, and the pain was front and center. As the body was rotated over and positioned on the backboard, Lincoln caught sight of the blood and all the damage to Jessie. His eyes rolled up in his head, and he toppled to the ground once again.

It took five people to transfer Jessie up the mountain and another half hour to get to the ambulance. Lincoln recovered enough to walk on his own with the group back to the ambulance. He was put in the front seat as they prepared Jessie for transport. Two IVs were started, a splint was placed on his broken leg, and a huge bandage was placed on his abdomen.

The transport to the hospital was another hour. Jessie was stable the entire time but in significant pain. He remained in the hospital for nearly two weeks. It took time to get all the small splinters and sufficient healing of the stomach. The initial surgery removed the piece of tree from his abdomen and cleaned it out as best as possible. The leg required surgery to place a metal plate to stabilize the leg.

Fortunately, he did not require an amputation. However, his ATV accident was serious, and he was lucky to have survived. Lincoln loved every minute of his ride-along and signed up for two others. Once he graduated high school, he planned on studying to become a doctor..

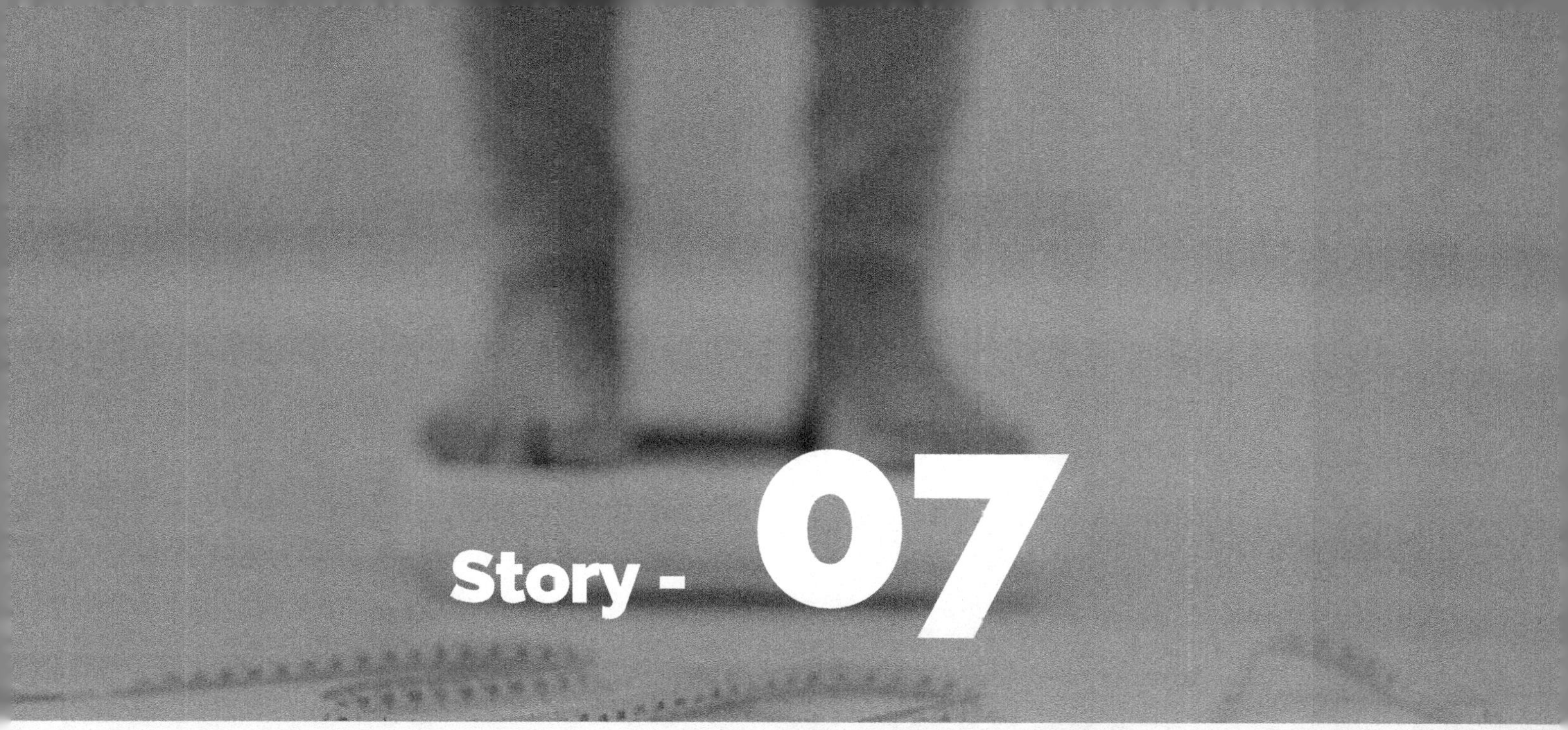

Story - 07

Are You Calling Me Fat?

As I was finishing up an exam with one patient in one room, I heard my next patient screaming and screaming in the next. Walking down the hall, it became clear that the patient did not appreciate what the nurse was trying to do. The patient kept asking, "Are you calling me fat?"

Nurse Collins, one of my more experienced nurses, must've also heard the shrieking, and she was already at the door, knocking and entering. Nurse Avery was striding out of the same room by the time I arrived. She was distraught and in tears.

I asked, "What's going on in there? Are you alright?"

Nurse Avery shook her head, and I walked with her for a few steps to get some privacy.

Nurse Avery shook as she said, "Ms. Ferguson became so upset when I checked her weight when she first arrived. I didn't know it would set her off. She has gained more than twenty pounds since her last appointment, six months ago."

"That's a substantial weight gain."

"That's what I was thinking. I asked her if she felt she was eating more or if it were possible that she could be pregnant. She bit off my head and screamed how she had found the right way to prevent pregnancy. I thought I calmed her down, and she admitted that she has been insecure because of her weight gain. She said she noticed it last week. She blew up again when I asked if she has been feeling sick in the morning."

"It's fine," I said. "You were just trying to help her. I'll go have a chat with her."

Nurse Avery smiled appreciatively and went to take a break. I returned to the door and found that Mrs. Ferguson was yelling again, this time at Nurse Collins. I knocked and entered the room.

"Hello, Ms. Ferguson, it's Doctor Maas. How are you doing today?"

She replied, "How do you think I'm doing?"

"Not well, by the sounds of things."

"I've never been so humiliated."

"I'm sorry that you're upset at my nurses' questions. They were just trying to get a little medical information before I came in to see you. Trust me. They were not trying to humiliate you."

"Well... a lot of those questions are about my weight. I'm very sensitive about how I look."

"I apologize again. I completely understand." I pulled out her chart and sat on a chair close to her. Nurse Collins took a few steps back, but stayed in the room. Opening her chart, I reviewed her previous weights, vitals, and complaints for the last few years. "I'm sorry that the questions made you feel uncomfortable. We are definitely not calling you fat. But these are questions we ask everyone when there's a change in the vitals. If it had been your blood pressure, our questions would have been related to your heart and such. Your weight six months ago was 127 pounds, and today you are 150 pounds. We just want to make sure there's nothing that we need to be aware of."

"But honestly," Mrs. Ferguson replied. "Talking about a girl's weight is a sensitive subject."

"I totally get that," I replied. "But there are things like Endocrine problems, Thyroid, Diabetes and such that could be associated with weight gain."

"What kind of thyroid problems?" she asked.

"Metabolism or the breakdown in food is largely affected by your thyroid. There are enzymes released from the thyroid that can cause it to speed up and slow down if they aren't released as they should. In cases like Hypothyroidism, your metabolism and other things can be affected by the lack of hormones. It's just one of the possible causes of your weight gain."

"Does there have to be something wrong with me?"

"No," I said quickly. "Not necessarily. Weight gain can be caused by stress, lack of exercise, lack of motivation, and other things. Have you felt you have been eating more than usual? Have you been getting less exercise?"

Ms. Ferguson had calmed down considerably. As was often the case, patients were more willing to answer questions with the doctor in the room. She even asked a few of her own. She admitted, "I have been eating a little more than usual. A few months ago, I had some stomach issues, and I thought I had an ulcer. I was nauseous every morning, but as the day went on, I started to feel better."

"When is the last time you felt nauseous?"

"A few weeks ago."

I nodded. "Is there any diabetes that runs in your family?"

She shook her head. "I don't think so. My parents and siblings are pretty healthy. They aren't overweight, and my grandparents are the same."

"It looks like you're turning twenty-two in the next few weeks."

"I am excited about my birthday."

"Do you smoke or drink?"

"I smoke about a half pack of cigarettes a day and drink maybe three or four times a week. I don't get drunk that often. It has been at least a few months."

"Thank you for that information. Were there other reasons that you came into the clinic today?"

"My period has been off the last few months. I get a little spotting every now and then. I'm usually pretty regular, but I was wondering if I should get an IUD or get on some birth control to help regulate my periods. I'm not good at taking the pill."

"Are you sexually active?"

"Yes. I live with my boyfriend, and we have a healthy relationship."

"Do you use protection?"

Her face went slightly pink. "Most of the time."

I nodded and wrote down a few things in my chart.

Mrs. Ferguson asked, "What do you think, Doctor Maas?"

"My recommendation is that we do some blood work and a pregnancy test. We can check for diabetes and thyroid issues and make sure everything else is going alright."

"I'm totally certain that I'm not pregnant."

"That may be true, but in order to be considered for an IUD, we must do a pregnancy test."

"Whatever," Mrs. Ferguson replied. "I guess I need to pee in a cup."

"Yes. Nurse Collins will take you to the bathroom. Afterward, she will take you down the hall to our phlebotomist. We'll get some blood and meet you back in here in a few minutes." Turning to Nurse Collins, I asked, "Can you show Ms. Ferguson the way to the bathroom."

"Sure, doctor."

Ms. Ferguson said, "You can call me Kelly."

I nodded.

Kelly was back in her room twenty minutes later. She sat on the exam table when nurse Collins and I walked in. I asked, "Can I do a quick exam?"

Kelly shrugged.

I listened to her heart, lungs, stomach, and did a general exam. She appeared healthy and strong. She had no other obvious signs of thyroid or diabetes. I asked, "Can I have the nurse check your blood sugar right now? This can help us understand if you have diabetes."

"I guess."

Her blood sugar was 87, and her blood pressure remained normal. Nurse Collins told her the results.

I said, "Well. We think we know what's going on. Of course, the lab work will take a few days, but we still have a pretty clear picture."

"Is there something wrong with me?" asked Kelly.

"Not-at-all," I replied. "Your blood pressure and blood sugar are normal. But we are confident that you are pregnant. The pregnancy test was positive."

"No way," Kelly replied. "That's not possible."

Nurse Collins pulled out the pregnancy test and showed it to her.

Kelly kept repeating, "Not possible."

"We also have this machine that can listen to the heart rate of your baby. Will you let us see if we can hear a heartbeat?"

"I guess," Kelly said, slightly in shock.

Nurse Collins brought in a machine and had Kelly lay down. She pulled up her shirt to reveal her belly. Some lubrication was placed on the skin. "If it's too early in the pregnancy, we can't hear anything, so we will see."

Nurse Collins placed the machine, and quickly the baby's heart rate was heard. The whooshing sound was quick and strong.

Tears began to fill in Kelly's eyes.

"I'm sure this is a lot to process," I said.

Kelly continued shaking her head. "I just can't believe this is happening to me. I must be one of the people where rare things happen to. I've heard that even with the pill or condoms, you can still get pregnant."

I said, "Earlier, you said that you sometimes forget to use protection."

"That's not what I meant. In the past, I have forgotten to take my pills. Those are hard to remember. But, for the past six months, my form of birth control has been smoking. My boyfriend and I smoke five cigarettes each before and after any sexual activity."

I shared a glance with my nurse. I hesitantly asked, "Why do you do that?"

"We've all heard the commercials. I also have talked with a lot of my friends, and they tell me that smoking can cause you to become infertile. It's the best way to prevent getting pregnant."

I had to cover my mouth quickly. When I dared to speak, I said, "Preventing pregnancy and being infertile are two different things. I see how that might be confusing. Infertility is an inability to get pregnant. Things like condoms and birth control prevent fertile women from getting pregnant. Smoking may cause infertility in a bad way, like an unwanted side effect, but it shouldn't be used as birth control."

Kelly shook her head. "It seems like the same thing."

Nurse Collins added, "It's not honey. Lots of women who smoke get pregnant. Infertility only happens in a small number of people who smoke. It is called an adverse effect."

"Whatever," Kelly replied. "How far along am I?"

"At least six or seven weeks, but it could be more."

"How do we tell?"

"An ultrasound."

We had a lot more explaining to do. She had several misconceptions about other things tied to pregnancy and women's health. We performed an ultrasound and ordered more blood work, an OBGYN visit, and a follow-up. Turned out she was twenty-two weeks pregnant.

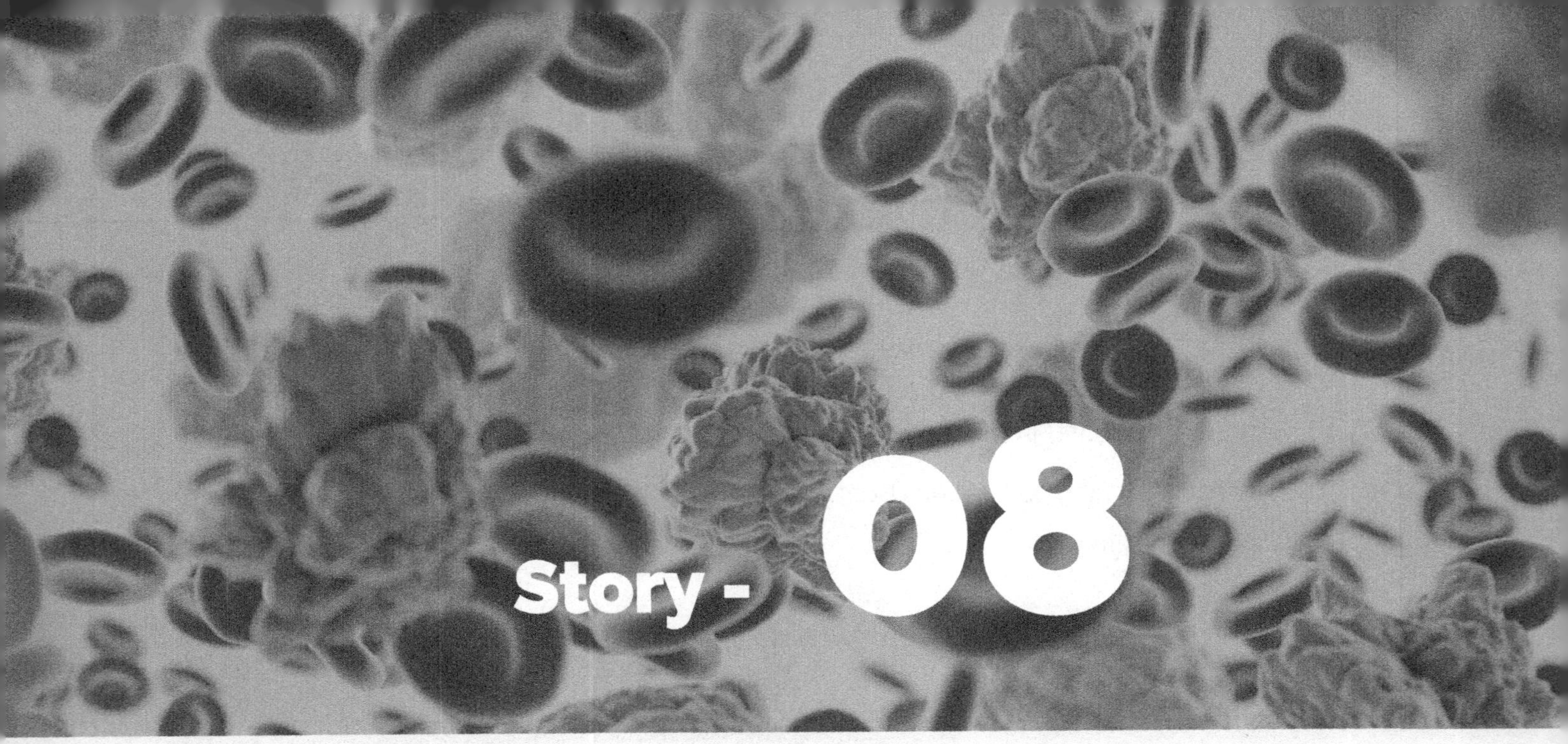

Worst Case of Misdiagnosed Acne Ever

We had a young boy that came into the emergency room with his mom. He was about seventeen, and his mom reported he had a bad case of acne. He had been put into a trauma room, and a nurse was sent to check him in. Before nurse Dan went into the room, he pulled me aside and showed me the complaint.

I asked, "Why would someone bring their child into the ER for acne?"

Nurse Dan replied, "I bet this will be a five-minute visit or less. One of the doctors will explain that acne is not life-threatening and can be taken care of through topical treatment, and if it gets bad, they can see a dermatologist."

I said, "There's a full moon out. I bet this is going to be a bit harder than that."

He walked away and added, "You just jinked it."

Ten minutes later, I heard someone screaming down the hall. I left the nursing station and found a woman hurrying around the hospital, calling for a doctor.

"Can I help you?" I asked.

"Are you a doctor?"

"No. But I can go find one. Tell me what is going on."

The mom explained that she was really concerned about her son. The nurse that had been in the room was asking too many questions, and the doctor had yet to arrive. She left the room and began searching for someone. Suddenly, she started jogging ahead of me, screaming, "Help. I need a doctor. My son is dying."

I followed her, trying to calm her. When I caught up to her, I said, "Listen. I know where the doctor is. I'll bring you to your room and go find them."

As we walked back to her son's room, she explained that he had severe acne on his arms. It had been getting worse the last few months. The acne on his face and back was far less noticeable. She reported that the same thing happened to one of his cousins. He had these sores on his arms, and when she had asked him, he had said it was acne. Another cousin on the opposite side of the family had required more advanced acne treatment. She had started looking up acne treatments online and heard of something called Accutane.

"I just know that if we can start him on that medication today, he will do better."

We arrived at her son's room just as Nurse Dan stepped out. I said, "This is Mrs. Schaffer, and she's the mother of your patient. She's really worried about her son's acne, and she's requesting that he starts treatment right away."

"I'm not sure that we are dealing with acne. We will likely need to run some tests and see if something more is going on."

"What? Of course, it's acne. My son's cousin had the same thing. Maybe this is just the worst case of acne you've ever seen, and you aren't sure how to treat it." Mrs. Chaffer added, "I'm telling you, if you start Accutane, he'll start feeling better in no time."

I watched as Nurse Dan's eyes enlarged, and a look of surprise crossed his face. He said, "Accutane is a very special medication however, it has lots of side effects. Treatment is the doctor's decision. If Accutane is approved, we'll need to run several blood tests to confirm that he's a candidate."

"Thank you for listening to me," she said.

"No problem."

I said, "Thanks Dan. I'll drop off Mrs. Schaffer."

As I entered the room, I was shocked to see the condition of Mrs. Schaffer's son. He was shaking, pale, and covered in clothing. Despite the layers of clothing, he was shivering. His eyes were closed, and he was stuffed under the blankets. The worse part was the extremely foul smell in the room, like decaying skin.

I asked, "When did the acne start?"

"About three or four months ago."

"He looks like he's freezing. Have we checked a temperature?"

"The first nurse said it was like one-hundred and three degrees."

"That's pretty elevated."

"It's probably from the sunburn. He hasn't reacted as well as I was hoping to the sunlight. I thought he was made of stronger stuff."

"What do you mean?"

"One of the recommended treatments for acne is sunlight. It's supposed to help with things like eczema and acne."

"How much sun are we talking about?"

Mrs. Chaffer pulled up the arm sleeves of his son, and the redness was frightening. But there were also large sores on his arms that looked nothing like acne.

"What else have you tried?" I asked hesitantly.

Mrs. Schaffer sat in a chair and added, "After some topical creams that the first doctor gave me, we tried toothpaste and urine mixed together. We were about to try bleach."

"You're kidding."

"No. The Urea in urine plus toothpaste is really supposed to be anti-acne with antioxidants."

"I don't think that is how it works."

She stared directly at me and said, "I hope this hospital is willing to try holistic treatments in addition to Accutane."

"Urine is not holistic, and toothpaste really is effective inside the mouth."

"Show how much you know."

"Well. I will go ask the doctor to consider some holistic measures. But you still want Accutane, right?"

"Yes. My sister said that will help keep acne away permanently."

I left and found Nurse Dan already talking with Doctor Sydney. I joined the conversation just as Dan said, "His arms have nothing to do with acne. He has a serious infection, and I'm worried his mother is making things worse."

I added, "I'm also concerned. His mother told me that they put urine and toothpaste on his arms to help with the acne. After that, they've been using sunlight. He has a terrible sunburn. They want holistic options."

Dr. Sydney said, "Thanks for warning me. Let's go take a look."

Back in the trauma room, Dr. Sydney was doing her exam. Her poker face was much better than ours. Now that his shirt was off, there were significant burns on the chest, back, and arms. "How did he get so burned?" asked Dr. Sydney.

"I took him to a tanning booth and uncovered only his arms, chest, and back. I think that once his skin peels, it will help with his acne."

"It won't," said Dr. Sydney flatly. "This is a much more serious medical issue than acne. And although that might be an issue, there are more important things that we need to address."

Mrs. Schaffer stood and began gathering her things. "It is clear, after talking with the charge nurse, it was obvious that natural treatment isn't possible in this hospital. I think it is time for us to leave."

Dr. Sydney said, "That's not a good idea. Your son is very sick, and if you leave, that will be child endangerment. I'll have to call the police."

"Why would you?"

"He is extremely sick. If he doesn't get treatment soon, it could become life-threatening."

"What are you talking about?"

"You see, your son can't control his body temperature right now because of this infection and the sunburn. We need to get some lab work but start an IV and give him some general antibiotics until we know better. I think he'll feel better if we get him started on some treatment. If we don't, he's going to get much worse."

"Fine," Mrs. Schaffer said.

Nurse Dan started an IV and started some fluids. Mrs. Schaffer's son was given some oral antibiotics, but he struggled with swallowing. In total, he has seven large boils on both arms. He had some minimal acne on his face, chest, and back. This acne would be considered a normal severity for a teenage boy.

The lab work returned a few hours later, but Mrs. Schaffer's son was only feeling marginally better. He was no longer shaking, but he was still extremely dehydrated. The fluid had helped him to urinate, and we tested that as well.

Dr. Sydney entered the trauma room and said, "Well...we're definitely not dealing with acne. Accutane would be unhelpful in this case."

"What are you talking about?" She pointed to her son's arms and said, "Can't you see this cystic acne?"

Dr. Sydney pulled out a tablet and brought up pictures of acne, especially on the arms. Next, she showed her what cystic acne looks like. Me, Nurse Dan, and another nurse came into the room.

Mrs. Shaffer replied, "That's not what I found on the internet."

"Additionally," continued Dr. Sydney, "your son tested positive for heroin. He has been using it for a while. Those sores on his arms are from shooting up."

"Ah...no. My son doesn't do drugs."

"That's not what the blood work shows. And that's not the worst thing. By not properly treating the injection areas, these sites are now seriously infected. Your son will need IV antibiotics for the next few days. Additionally, we will need to watch his heart because it looks like he is at risk for sepsis."

"How long are we talking?"

"He's going to be in the hospital for a few days."

Dr. Sydney moved closer to her son and took a seat. She took out several needles with medications and a scalpel.

"What are you doing?"

"We need to drain these abscesses. Treatment will become far more successful if we do this."

The next hour was spent cutting into each abscess on both arms. Some were small, but three were gigantic. The smell was horrible, and Mrs. Schaffer left after just a few openings. There was so much purulent discharge that even I was impressed. This was the worst case of fake acne I had ever seen.

The next day, Mrs. Schaffer told me that she spoke with her sister-in-law, who confronted her son's cousin, and he admitted that he had shot up with him. They had been doing heroin together for three months.

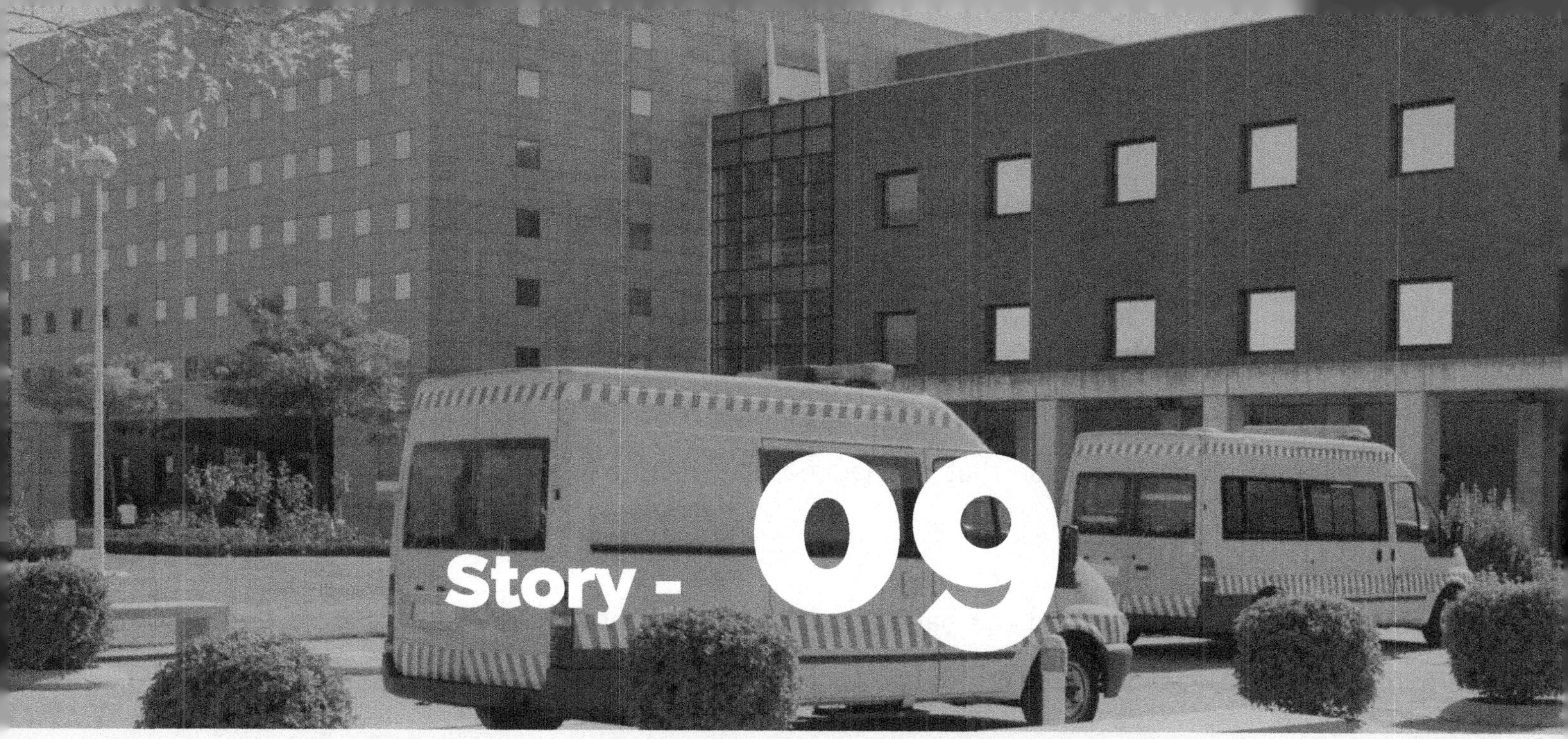

A Drop Off at the Hospital

Around two in the morning, our camera caught a man walking up from the street and into the ambulance bay at our Emergency Room. Suddenly, the man tripped and seemed to fall face-first onto the concrete. While lying there, he pulled out his phone and called 911. He told the dispatcher that he had been in a serious car accident the day before and that he was on his way to the hospital. The guy told the dispatcher that he was about to be dropped off at the hospital and couldn't walk. His friend had been driving last night, and he didn't want to get his friend in trouble. He hadn't been drinking, but his friend had been.

We, of course, didn't know about him falling or walking up to the hospital. The dispatcher called our nursing station, and we were sent out to the front of the hospital with a gurney. The man was lying on his back, reporting pain in his lower and mid-back. He said that he couldn't feel either of his legs. He was also worried that he might have a concussion and that he had split open his head and might have broken his left wrist.

The patient was quickly placed on a backboard, lifted to the gurney, and brought into the hospital and one of the trauma rooms. A few nurses were brought in to help, and I was in charge of the wound on his head. He had a gash on the top of his head that was jagged, thick, and bleeding profusely. The man was crying and screaming in severe pain.

Doctor Lee arrived and assessed the patient quickly. He was emotional and in pain, but he wasn't going through a life-and-death situation. But there was a lot that we didn't know.

"Mr. Oliver. I am Doctor Lee. Do you know where you are?"

"Am I having another seizure?" Mr. Oliver asked. "If not, I must be at the stadium."

"You are at the hospital. Do you remember getting dropped off? Do you remember a car accident?"

"Vaguely."

I was situated near the top of the gurney, where the head was bleeding as Dr. Lee was off to one side, trying to talk to the patient. I put pressure on the wound, but it kept bleeding. I went through several gauge dressings.

"Is pressure helping that cut?" asked Dr. Lee.

"No. I can't get it to stop right now."

"Wake up, Mr. Oliver," said the doctor. He rubbed at his chest and shoulders. The man's eyes were heavy and unfocused. "I'm going to fix your head first."

Mr. Oliver mumbled, "Please help me. I am in so much pain."

"When was the accident? You told the dispatcher it was a car accident."

"The night before last, I think. Maybe it was a few hours ago."

"Where you wearing a seat belt?"

"I wasn't, but my friend, the drive was. I just don't want him to get in trouble."

"I'm going to staple your head and send you for some scans on your back."

"Please put in stitches. I have a bad reaction to staples."

Dr. Lee began working on closing the head wound. An IV was placed by another nurse, and some pain medications were given. I helped gather supplies and adjust the light for Dr. Lee. It took about forty minutes to close the wound. It was really jagged, and there were some small pieces of rock removed from the wound.

Mr. Oliver was sent for CT imaging on his mid-back, neck, and lower back. However, two minutes after he arrived, he screamed that he was having a panic attack and needed Valium. He explained that he was claustrophobic and would not be able to relax. We needed him to be as still as possible. I've seen patients try to break their restraints while getting a CT. Valium was given.

Upon returning to the trauma room after the scan, he was crying and very emotional. He told me that his head was throbbing, he had some vision changes, and his eyes felt blurry. He thought he was going to vomit. I left to tell Dr. Lee.

Because of the large head laceration and his possible risks, he was next sent for an MRI. He was given some medications to stop him from throwing up. Again, shortly after he arrived, he complained about anxiety and was given Valium.

Immediately after getting out of the MRI, his pain was uncontrollable, and more pain medications were given. The CT exam results came back first, and he had some chronic findings that might have been made worse by the car accident, but nothing alarming was noted.

The patient was groggy when removed from his restraints following the CT results and fell asleep for a few hours. When he woke, he was starving. By this time, we knew the MRI did not show a brain bleed. Some food was brought in for Mr. Oliver. As he ate the last bite, he screamed that his wrist was hurting. He became animated and upset about his wrist.

He demanded, "What if we had been looking at the wrong place for my pain?"

He was sent for an X-ray.

After he had been in the ER for three hours, Dr. Lee returned. "Mr. Oliver. We feel very confident that you have no lasting injuries from the car accident. You may be sore for the next few days, but your back did not show a fracture or anything alarming. Your brain scan did not show a bleed, and there is no large concern for a severe concussion. Your wrist X-ray shows a previous fracture, but that is now healed, and you have some arthritis."

"Doctor. I hurt so bad. I can barely move my wrist."

"We will give you a few days of pain medications. We can give you a wrist brace. You need to go home and rest. Wear the splint for the next few days."

"What happens if I don't get better?"

"You can always return if something gets worse."

"What about a follow-up?"

"You can see your doctor in about a week or so to have the sutures removed from your head."

"Thank you, doctor, very much."

Mr. Oliver was discharged and left about twenty minutes later. He didn't have anyone who could come to get him, and a cab was called, and he was brought to the car door in a wheelchair.

An hour later, there was a phone call for Dr. Lee. When he picked it up, there was a doctor from a hospital across town on the other end.

"Hello, Dr. Lee. This is Dr. Rebecca Blanch. I am one of the ER physicians and wanted to talk to you about Mr. Oliver."

"Yes."

"The patient says that he was in a car accident last week and that you refused to see or treat him. He has a gaping wound on his head that needs sutures, and he says that he can't walk."

"Dr. Blanch. He left our ER an hour ago. We did multiple CT scans, MRI, wrist X-ray, and everything came back negative."

"He says that you guys kicked him out because he didn't have insurance. While he was leaving, he felt dizzy and fell and hit his head."

Dr. Lee countered by saying, "He told us that he was in a car accident, and I personally placed fourteen sutures in his head while here at the hospital. He has a jagged cut on the top of his head. It was a deep and complete laceration. We placed him on a backboard and did the full workup."

"What about the gushing cut on his forehead?"

"He left here in a wheelchair, and we saw him into a cab."

Dr. Blanch paused for a moment. "I think we are going to review our cameras. Will you do the same?"

"Certainly."

While looking at the footage from our cameras, we found that Mr. Oliver had walked up to the ambulance bay and tripped. We went further back and found him strolling down a street adjacent to the hospital. It did not appear that he was not wounded or injured at this point. As we followed him, we watched in horror as he ran head-first and dove into a pile of rocks. He hit his head extremely hard, and the man staggered when he stood, blood dripping onto his face and clothes. He struggled to walk the next few hundred feet to our parking lot and into the ambulance bay.

Dr. Blanch called back twenty minutes later, and they had found him arriving at the hospital in a taxi. He sat by a corner and used a knife to cut out the sutures placed by Dr. Lee. He next stood and started hitting his head into the wall until it was bleeding.

Mr. Oliver was confronted and admitted to self-sabotage because he couldn't afford the pills he was getting from the streets. Prices had gone up. He had gone to Walgreens and found a bottle of Aspirin and took the entire thing before deciding to go to the hospital. That was the reason his head wound kept bleeding.

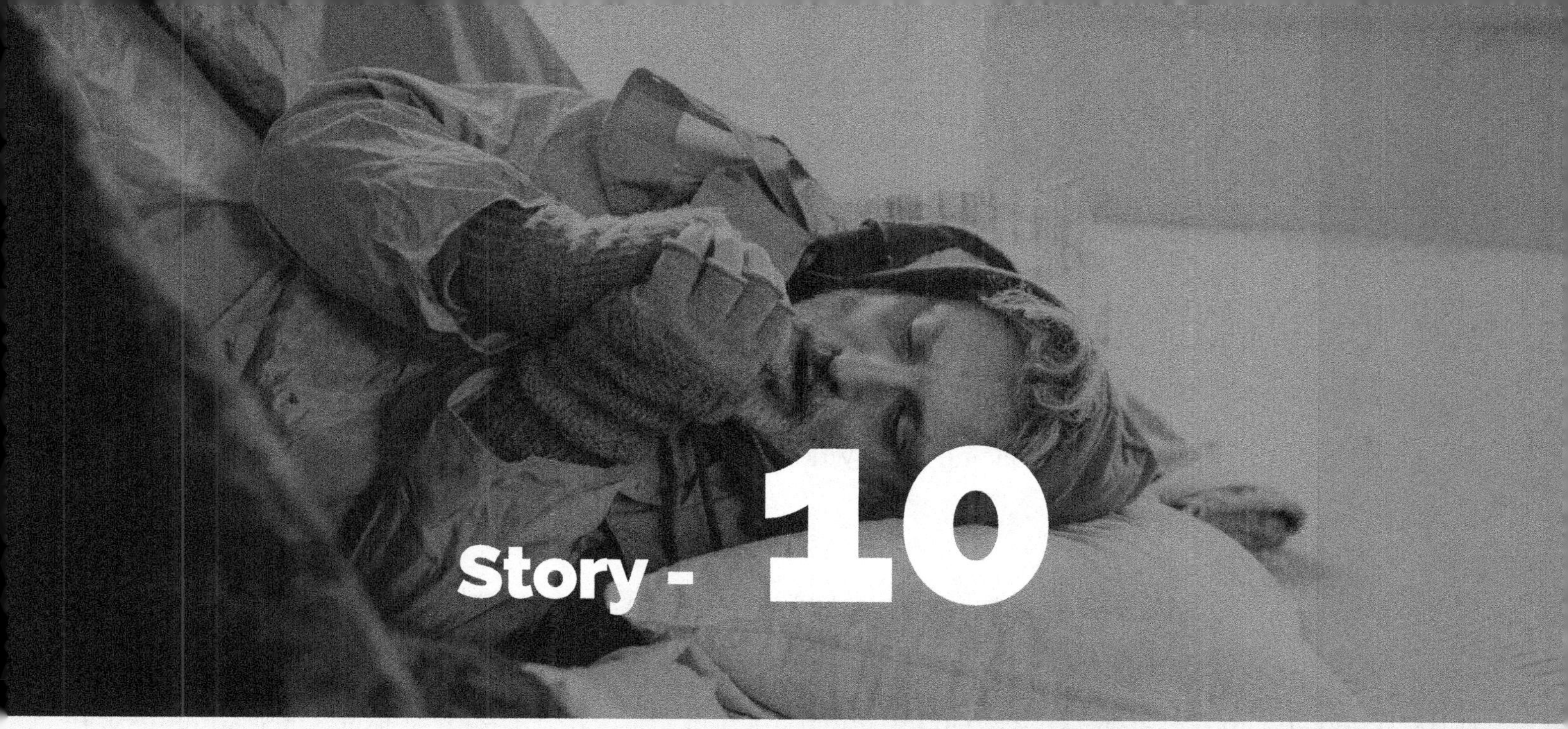

Story - 10

Hypothermia and a Hidden Treasure

Working on the ambulance, we see some pretty crazy things. Some are more traumatizing than others. Luckily this one time, I experienced a positive result with a funny side-story. It was late at night, and the temperature was dropping fast. A snowstorm was coming in from the west, and we were getting some lake effect. The temperature was expected to drop below zero for the first time all year.

We had been on two calls at two different houses that turned out to be nothing serious. This was good because that meant we had a break from some food. We stopped at a local diner that our crew frequented a lot. I simply love their potpie. It is a well-known place, and it was busy, but we were ushered to our usual spot. There are three of us on our crew. Drew and Cindy were a year or two more experienced than I was. But our team worked well together.

Cindy might take the lead, and another call would be Drew or myself. Halfway through eating, our ambulance and another were called to the local park to help with some of the homeless. When the temperature drops, the homeless look for a better place to shelter for the night. If they are lucky, they can find room at one of the dozens of shelters in the city. The number of beds is always limited, so other places are under bridges, parks, inside cars left open, abandoned buildings, and wherever they might find refuge for the night. We were called to a homeless camp at Memorial Park.

As we drove to the location, we received updated information. There had been a fight, and the police had been called. However, during the investigation, a man was found unconscious and not breathing. We arrived at the scene and immediately were led in the right direction. Police had already started chest compressions. It appeared that the man was found in a tent by himself.

The three of us each had a different responsibility. I wrote down the necessary information and received additional data from the other two paramedics, officers, and bystanders over the next fifteen minutes. The man appeared to be in his fifties or sixties but guessing the age of someone who is homeless is just as much luck as experience. An IV was started, pads were placed to check the heart, and vitals were done. It quickly became apparent that the homeless man was alive, breathing, and had a reasonable heart rate. Contrary to the first report, he was breathing and calm. For some reason, we couldn't wake him up. We used Narcan and ammonia to elicit a response, but nothing.

The patient was moved to a gurney and strapped down. We placed all the machines and IV lines correctly and started piling on blankets. The man was suffering from hypothermia and potentially something more serious. He was quickly loaded onto the ambulance, and I drove. This situation was an emergency but not necessarily life-threatening. We promptly went to the nearest hospital. We unloaded the patient and walked into the hospital. We were quickly assigned to a room and helped transfer the patient from our gurney to the hospital bed.

Rebecca, a nurse we knew well, came into the exam room. Drew and Cindy stepped out, and I helped as much as possible. I was shocked to discover that the man's jeans were soaking wet and nearly frozen. It was as if he had walked in water before he lay down. His socks and shoes were equally wet.

She began cutting off the clothing we couldn't easily remove. She took off a thick jacket and a button-up shirt. These were mostly dry. She was forced to cut off the man's socks and pants. It was clear he had not bathed in weeks. The aroma of the room became rancid. Rebecca positioned EKG leads, and more testing was done. She used the same IV line that we had done as it was still working.

"We need some heating blankets," said Dr. Johnson, who stepped in for a moment.

First, Rebecca started drying off the man's legs. Using some towels, she quickly dried off each leg and foot. She lifted them and rubbed at the skin, which was whiter than pink, especially below the waist.

"Bring in a hemodialysis machine, just in case," added Dr. Johnson. "Let's send out some blood work—if we can get it."

Rebecca nodded, and I took over the drying process. Rebecca went to the opposite arm as the IV and pulled out some blood for testing.

Jackie, a med-tech, brought in heating blankets to the room, and it didn't take long for the homeless man to be covered entirely.

The next step was for us to wait. Being paramedics, we always take opportunities that are presented. We stopped by the cafeteria to grab some food. We spend a decent amount of time driving around or at the hospital. Even between calls, we catch up with friends at this hospital. We didn't get a chance to finish our meal, so we grabbed some snacks.

Drew and Cindy remained outside the room, but I was curious about how this process would turn out. A hemodialysis machine would remove blood, warm it up, and return it to the body. It is only used in severe circumstances, and fortunately, this homeless man did not need it.

He remained unconscious for an hour, but his vitals remained stable. His heart rate was strong. It was as if he was having trouble waking up, but Dr. Johnson and Rebecca didn't feel he was in any immediate danger.

The man woke up just before we were about to leave. We hadn't received our next call, but it was time to get back out on the streets. We still had three or four hours left of our shift. I stopped by his room, and Rebecca hurried in and began checking his vitals.

"Where am I?" the man asked.

"At the hospital."

"Why? Did I get injured?" The man's mouth was dry, and his voice was raw.

"The police found you, and you were unconscious. Do you remember what happened?"

Jackie brought in some warm coffee.

After a few sips, the man said, "I was chased and ran through the park. I had to hide in the river so that those boys wouldn't hurt me."

"What boys?" asked Rebecca.

"I don't know who they were. They just laughed at me."

"Then what happened?" Rebecca asked.

"I made my way back to my tent and collapsed."

I added, "That's where the police found you. I am one of the paramedics that found you and brought you to the hospital."

"Thank you, young man."

"No problem, Mr..."

"—Mr. Conaway," the man replied.

I shook his hand and I left. I updated Drew and Cindy about the good outcome. We drove off and responded to another call.

While we were driving an hour later or so, my phone began ringing. It was Rebecca from the hospital.

After greeting each other, Rebecca said, "You're not going to believe what happened."

"Is Mr. Conaway okay?"

"Yes. He's fine. Resting comfortably."

"Good. Tell me what happened."

Rebecca continued, her voice animated, "Thirty minutes after you left, Mr. Conaway asked about his clothing. I told him that we had to cut the pants and socks. He asked about his shirt and jacket. I didn't know where they had gone."

I said, "I remember Jackie coming in and taking all the clothing."

"Makes sense. That's what I thought had happened."

"She was going to destroy them."

"Exactly. That's what I told him. I explained that we had plenty of extra clothing to give him. He wanted to know specifically about his jacket. I told him that it was likely destroyed. He went crazy. He started screaming and shouting and tried to get out of his bed. He went nuts. I didn't know what to do."

"Because of his jacket?" I asked. "I don't remember it being top quality or anything."

"Me neither. I couldn't calm him down, and he kept screaming for his jacket. I told him that I would look for it. Luckily, I caught Jackie just a minute or two before she was going to incinerate the jacket. I retrieved it and brought it back to Mr. Conaway. When I walked in the room, he hugged it like it was his long-lost friend."

"Are you messing with me?"

"No. I finally got the truth out of him. At first, I thought it had sentimental value. There was fifteen thousand dollars sewed into the lining."

"No way."

"He showed me. There were four or five pins on the inside that, when he removed them, I could see dozens and dozens of different types of bills. I didn't count it, but..."

I stated, "He had fifteen thousand dollars stuffed in his jacket, and he's living on the streets."

"He said he rarely uses the money, but it's for an emergency," replied Rebecca. "And it helps keep him warm."

"That's hard to believe."

Rebecca said, "I would've never believed it had I not seen it."

"Why does he hide his money?"

"He said that he's afraid that they'll steal his coat if anyone else finds out."

I said, "He has good reason. I bet that would happen. Is he still getting better?"

"Yea. He'll be here for another few days. Might get some mild frostbite on his toes, but I think in time, he will be just fine.".

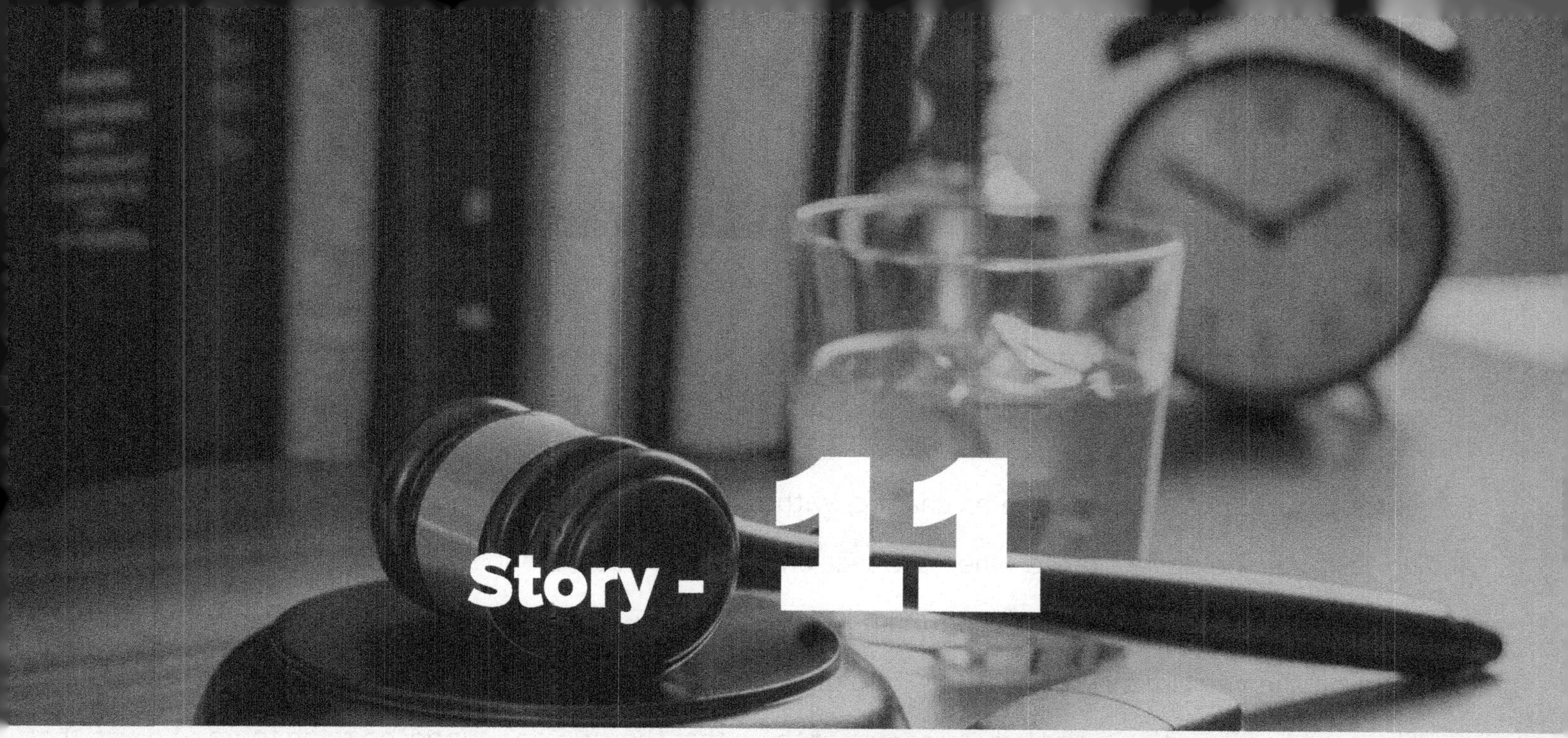

Story - 11

A DUI Patient for the Ages

As an ER doctor, I have come across many patients who have affected me over the years. This can be both a good and bad thing. When I went into the medical field, I had a lot of empathy and compassion toward my patients. That continues even to this day. However, I also have been battered with patients that lie, steal, manipulate, and return to the ER with the same complaint repeatedly. Over time, it gets difficult to see similar problems and results from the same patient repeatedly.

However, I am often reminded of the need for compassion and diligence in treating all of our patients. In the ER, we see a lot of similar types of injuries, self-injuries, self-destructive behavior, and much more. Balance with compassion is also important. Sometimes we have staff who become too involved with the patients, which can be problematic. Other times, there's not enough.

One night, Officer Marshall brought in a lady following a car accident. He described the scene when he arrived - she was attacking the person she had hit at a red light. It was a mess. The officer determined that the lady was driving under the influence. She was hallucinating, acting bizarrely, and not herself. He had no choice but to arrest her.

The witnesses described the scene as chaotic, with a lady crashing into the car in front of her. She wasn't driving fast, but she never braked when she rear-ended the vehicle stopped at a red light. After a minute or so, the lady exited her car and began pounding on the window of the car. At first, they thought the lady was checking on the vehicle, but she was talking gibberish. The two passengers came out of the car, and things quickly escalated from there. The lady screamed at them that they weren't supposed to be there. She said that they were trying to break into her house. She started hitting both people. The lady wasn't strong, but she "had a look in her eyes."

The officer arrived and quickly separated the two parties. It became clear that the lady was under the influence. The officer arrested her for simple battery and DUI. She was brought to the hospital to get a clearance before she was taken to jail. The lady was uncooperative on the way to the hospital, and she was confused and was handcuffed to the bed.

Hospital clearances often happen, maybe a few times a week. It could be for a DUI, after an arrest or car accident, and much more. Some of the individuals arrested are brought to the hospital with some of the craziest injuries.

As I walked to the patient's room, the officer said, "Good luck."

Entering the exam room, I found the patient was breathing hard as if she had been running a race. The nurse inside said, "She's starting to calm down."

"How old is she?"

"Seventy-eight."

The officer, and half the nursing staff, walked in a minute later. The officer said, "This is Mrs. Beverly. She used to be a schoolteacher and is the nicest person in the world."

I said, "You didn't tell me she was elderly and my neighbor. Why did you arrest her?"

"Doctor Ferguson. Telling you her age and who she is would have been far less fun. She just needs help."

"Officer Marshall, I know Mrs. Beverly quite well. She's good friends with my wife and children. She's the sweetest person in the world."

"I was shocked when I saw her attacking the people in the other car," Officer Marshall explained. "I had no idea what was happening."

Turning to one of the nurses in the room, I said, "Julie. Let's get some blood work. Start an IV, and we will probably have to get a CT scan." To the officer, I asked, "Could she have hit her head during the accident?"

"It's possible."

We watched Mrs. Beverly for the next four or five hours. She calmed down considerably and even slept some. It took a few hours, but we were able to get everything back from the blood work and CT scan. Almost everything was normal; at least, there weren't any alarming findings.

After Mrs. Beverly woke up, I went in to talk with her. I asked, "Do you know where you are?"

"At the hospital. You're Doctor Mike Ferguson. I taught your kids, and I live four or five houses down from you."

"That's right," I said. "What happened? Do you know why you are here?"

"I have no idea. Is everything alright?"

"You were in a car accident last night."

"A car accident?" Mrs. Beverly asked. She shook her head. "Not possible. I don't go out driving at night anymore. I have problems seeing in the dark. Since Benjamin passed away, I'm in bed by eight o'clock."

"I'm just telling you what happened."

"Why am I handcuffed to the bed?" Mrs. Beverly asked.

Officer Marshall stepped forward. "Nancy. You were driving last night, and you hit another car. You got out of the car and banged on the window. You were talking really weird and even hit the driver. Were you drinking last night?"

"I don't think so," Mrs. Beverly thundered. "You must be mistaken. I haven't had anything to drink in twenty years."

"Sorry. I had to ask. You weren't yourself last night."

"This doesn't seem right." Nancy Beverly shook her head. "Is this really happening to me? Is there something wrong with me, doctor?"

"I was worried after your accident, but your head CT scans were all normal. Your blood work was pretty normal."

"What do you mean - pretty normal?"

"Well," I said. "There were a few things that were unexpected."

"Like what?"

"You had both meth and marijuana in your system."

"What are you talking about? Methamphetamine and marijuana. I've never used either of those."

Nurse Julie said, "We checked a few times. It's true."

"Impossible," Mrs. Beverly said. Looking up at Doctor Ferguson, she asked, "Can you explain how all of this is possible?"

"Not really. Do you smoke at all?"

"Of course, I don't."

Officer Marshall said, "Sometimes you can eat something with Meth and Marijuana."

"Like what?"

"Gummy bears, cookies, hard candies, and other edibles."

"You're talking nonsense. Where would I get any of those things?"

They left Mrs. Beverly alone for several minutes to gather her thoughts.

Officer Marshall said, "This morning, I spoke to the other individuals involved, and they know Mrs. Beverley and aren't pressing charges. We aren't going to take her to jail, but she acted pretty weird last night. She seems to be better right now."

I said, "Some people have weird reactions to marijuana and meth. I'm hoping that's what happened here. I can't explain it right now, but she likely consumed something."

"I have to be going," Officer Marshall added. "My shift is over. Let me know."

Early the next morning, the new staff was about to arrive at the hospital. The three children of Mrs. Beverly walked through the doors, and the situation was explained to them. They were told that she wasn't going to be arrested but that they needed to keep a close eye on her. Each of them agreed. One of her sons appeared less surprised by the situation than the rest. The rest of the family was ushered out to the waiting area, and Johnathan remained in his mom's room.

When everyone was gone, Jonathan asked, "Did Eric drop by to see you yesterday?"

Mrs. Beverly responded, "My grandson? Yes. I love it when he comes to see me. He brought me some brownies. I think I ate a few."

"Oh boy," Jonathan said. "He's gotten in trouble a few times. He has been creative in his baking skills."

"What does that mean?" Mrs. Beverly asked.

"I think he brought you the wrong brownies. I'm going to kill that kid."

Sure enough. Eric had agreed to make the brownies for some friends for a party that night. The problem was that he brought the wrong ones to his grandmother's house. Eric was grounded for the entire summer and was fortunate that he didn't go to jail himself. Both cars were fixed, and the situation was resolved. Mrs. Beverly laughs about it to this day..

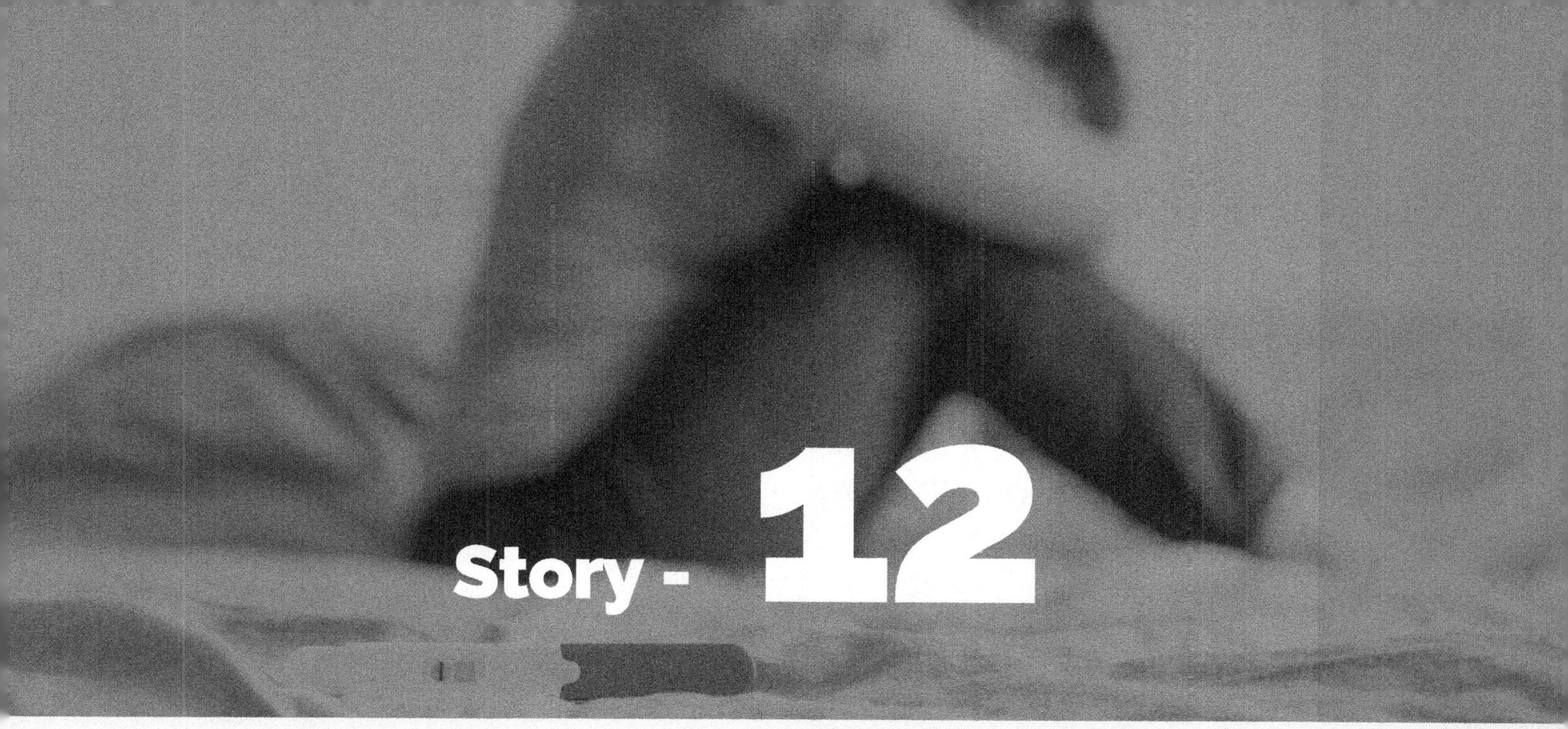

Story - 12

Frustrations of Trying to Get Pregnant

A female patient came into our clinic requesting some information, general testing, and a specific workup for infertility. She was in her thirties and had been with her partner for three years. They wanted to have children, but thus far, had been unsuccessful. She was here, secretly, without her partner because she was worried that the infertility was her fault.

She had spent a fair amount of time on the internet researching PCOS, Diabetes, and several other genetic causes of infertility. She was overwhelmed, anxious, and had plenty of self-pity. It had taken her months to get the courage to come to our clinic.

The nurse checked her in and went over the basics of her health, medications, and family history. There were no reports of any infertility in her parents, grandparents, or siblings. She was not on any concerning medications and had no significant medical history.

After she was arranged in her room, I went to see her. She was distraught and uncomfortable. After introducing myself as Dr. Pamala Larson, we began the visit.

"Hello, Gretchen. I was told by my nurse that you are here with some very personal questions and concerns."

"Yes, Dr. Larson. My partner and I are struggling to have children."

"Have you ever been pregnant before? Maybe a miscarriage or something."

"No, nothing."

"Have you always wanted to have children?"

"No. For the longest time, I didn't. A year after I married my first husband, we started trying, but we were never successful. Two years later, it seemed like every one of our fights was centered around not getting pregnant. He became somewhat verbally aggressive. He blamed me over and over again, and he finally left me."

"That's terrible. Did you guys get checked out for infertility during your marriage?"

"Oh, no. He was far too proud."

"How long has it been since you have seen anyone for your female health?"

"It's been a while," Gretchen admitted.

"I think we should start with a regular physical exam and a pap smear. Does that sound okay?"

"I guess. It has been several years since my last lady exam."

Her physical exam was normal. She was overly uncomfortable getting undressed before the exam, and Dr. Larson left the room for a few minutes to let her get undressed. She did the same after the exam was finished.

"How does everything look?" she asked once Dr. Larson stepped back into the room.

"Did you think that something was amiss?"

"Not really," she said quickly. "I haven't really ever thought about it before. My ex-husband always blamed me, and I started believing it recently. I just was worried that maybe my partner, and I couldn't have children because there might be something wrong with me."

"From that standpoint, there is nothing wrong."

"Then what could it be?"

"There are several things that can cause infertility. We should run some tests, some blood work, and maybe an ultrasound. We can meet again in a week or so, and next time, maybe you can bring in your partner and we could run some tests as well."

"What kind of tests?"

"Hormones are pretty important to pregnancy, and there are several other things that we need to look at."

"Oh, I don't want to hear about that. I get grossed out when I think about that stuff."

"What do you mean?"

"I hate the idea of donating blood or any needle sticks. I would rather not talk about hormones and the other stuff."

"If we want to help you, it is imperative that we find a cause. Do you still want to get tested for infertility?"

"Yes," Gretchen said after a slight pause. "This is something that is important to me. I want to know the truth."

"Alright. It's a plan. Let's get you tested. I've ordered the lab work, and you can get it done at the clinic down the street. I'll call you back in a few days, and we can schedule an appointment for a follow-up.

Ten days later, Gretchen was back in the clinic. She had gotten the blood work done, and earlier this morning, the ultrasound was completed. Dr. Larson had looked at the results of both. Gretchen was anxiously waiting, fearing the worst.

She admitted to the nurse checking her vitals that she was far more nervous about the blood work results than she had been for the pap smear. She was also alone.

"Well," said Dr. Larson upon entering. "Thanks for coming back for this follow-up. It looks like everything came back normal. You definitely have normal hormones, and there were plenty of eggs from the blood work that we got. The ultrasound was normal as well."

"That's a relief," replied Gretchen.

"I was hoping to see your partner today, to do some testing on them."

"Yea. Like my ex-husband, my partner is proud, and she doesn't think that the infertility is her fault."

"Her fault?" asked the doctor. "Is your partner female?"

"Yes. I know it is unconventional for two parents to be women, but I've heard that is happening more and more."

"You both being women is not really the issue."

Gretchen asked, "Then what is the problem?"

"Who is hoping to become pregnant?"

"At first it was me, but now, we both want to be pregnant. It's actually a little competition between the two of us to see who can become pregnant first."

Dr. Larson sat across from Gretchen, trying to assess the situation. Delicacy and tact were required at this point. "Why do you think that this is an infertility thing?"

"We tried so many times, and neither of us has gotten pregnant. Initially, we agreed that I would be the one to get pregnant, but after we failed so many times, my partner was willing to try. We've honestly been attempting for almost nine months straight. When my partner heard about my problems with my first husband, it became natural to think that it was infertility and my fault."

"Okay," Dr. Larson said. "This is going to come out wrong, but you understand how a woman gets pregnant, right?"

"Sexual activity. You have a sperm and an egg, and they combine, and voila!"

"Okay, yes. But if you are engaging in sexual activity between two women, there is no sperm involved, and it would be impossible to get pregnant."

Gretchen's face reddened. "Oh. Now I understand. I completely forgot to mention that we are using some sperm from a male friend of my partner. He agreed to help us get pregnant. He donates it a few times a week, and we keep it in the fridge. It just doesn't seem to be working."

Dr. Larson sat slightly more straight in her chair. "Okay. Now I'm getting a clearer picture."

"You do?" Gretchen asked.

"I don't think the problem is infertility but the process. For either of you to become pregnant, you need to have some help through the ART program or assisted reproductive technology. In this case, someone in my clinic would introduce the sperm through a tube directly into the uterus."

"We were trying to do the same thing."

"I agree," said Dr. Larson kindly. "But the process you were trying is nearly impossible."

"Are you sure?"

"Yes. We do this all the time."

"Even with two women?"

"Of course."

Gretchen and her partner came back to the clinic the following week for the procedure. They were receptive and easy to work with. They were so excited about the possibilities of a new family. Everything went smoothly, and Dr. Larson was pleased to learn that Gretchen tested positive for pregnancy a few weeks later. The next few months went as smoothly as possible, and when the time came, she gave birth to a baby girl..

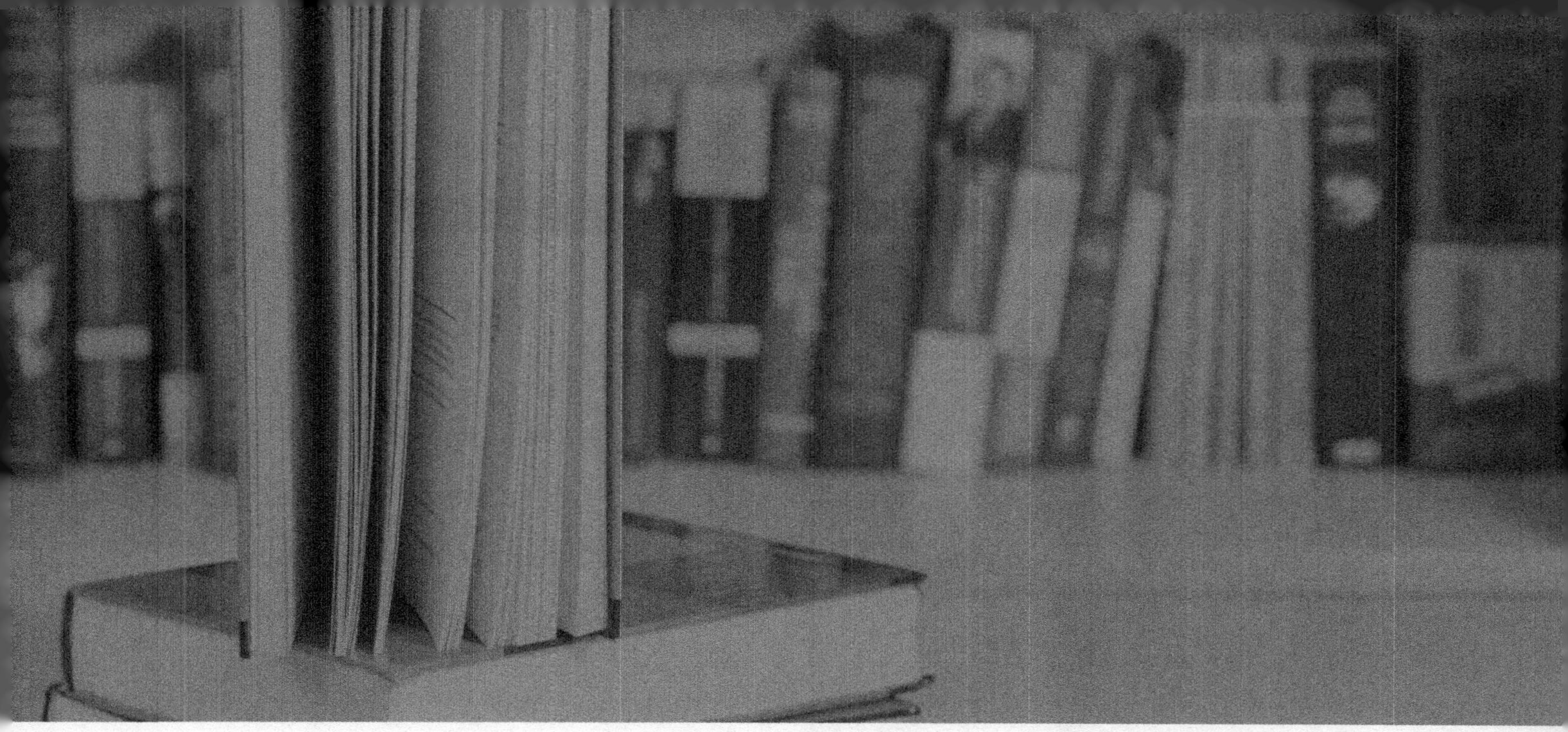

Tales of the Exam Room Collection

Check out our other Volumes:

Crazy Medical Stories: **Tales of the Exam Room - Volume 1**

10 Short stories about the crazy world of Medicine. These stories have taken years to collect, understand, and write. Author Scott Kemp has worked tirelessly to bring for you this entertaining perspective of the patient and medical staff relationship. Each story brings about a greater clarity into the delicate choices presented day in and day out.

https://www.amazon.com/Crazy-Medical-Stories-Tales-Exam/dp/1736159844/ref=tmm_pap_swatch_0?_encoding=UTF8&qid=1618501286&sr=8-2

Medical Horror Stories: **Tales of the Exam Room - Volume 2**

10 Short stories about the crazy world of Medicine. In Vol 2, we continue exploring the astonishing world of medicine as we discover some of the unpredictable situations between patients and medical professionals. Often, like a law of nature, when something can go wrong, it does. But the outcome is rarely as you expect it.

https://www.amazon.com/Medical-Horror-Stories-Tales-Exam/dp/1736159860/ref=sr_1_5?dchild=1&keywords=Tales+of+the+Exam+room&qid=1613685694&sr=8-5

Medical Stories While Incarcerated: **Tales of the Exam Room - Volume 3**

12 Short stories about the crazy world of Medicine. Medicine happens in all shapes and forms. We are excited to present these stories centered around medical stories that happen in jails and prisons. But beware, these stories are a step or two more graphic than our previous stories. We have a long-standing love for medicine and some of the unimaginable situations that patients and medical professionals find themselves in.

https://www.amazon.com/Tales-Exam-Room-Medical-Incarcerated/dp/B08NYTQ6GX/ref=sr_1_4?dchild=1&keywords=Tales+of+the+Exam+Room&qid=1606499209&sr=8-4

Scary Medical Stories: **Tales of the Exam Room - Volume 4**

12 Short stories in Vol. 4 that takes a look into the extreme side of medicine. This includes a boy getting hit in the chest with a ball, relenting episodes of vomiting, and much more. This set of stories helps you appreciate the importance and impact of medical professionals in difficult situations.

Scary Medical Stories: Tales of the Exam Room Volume 4: Kemp, Scott: 9781954814059: Amazon.com: Books

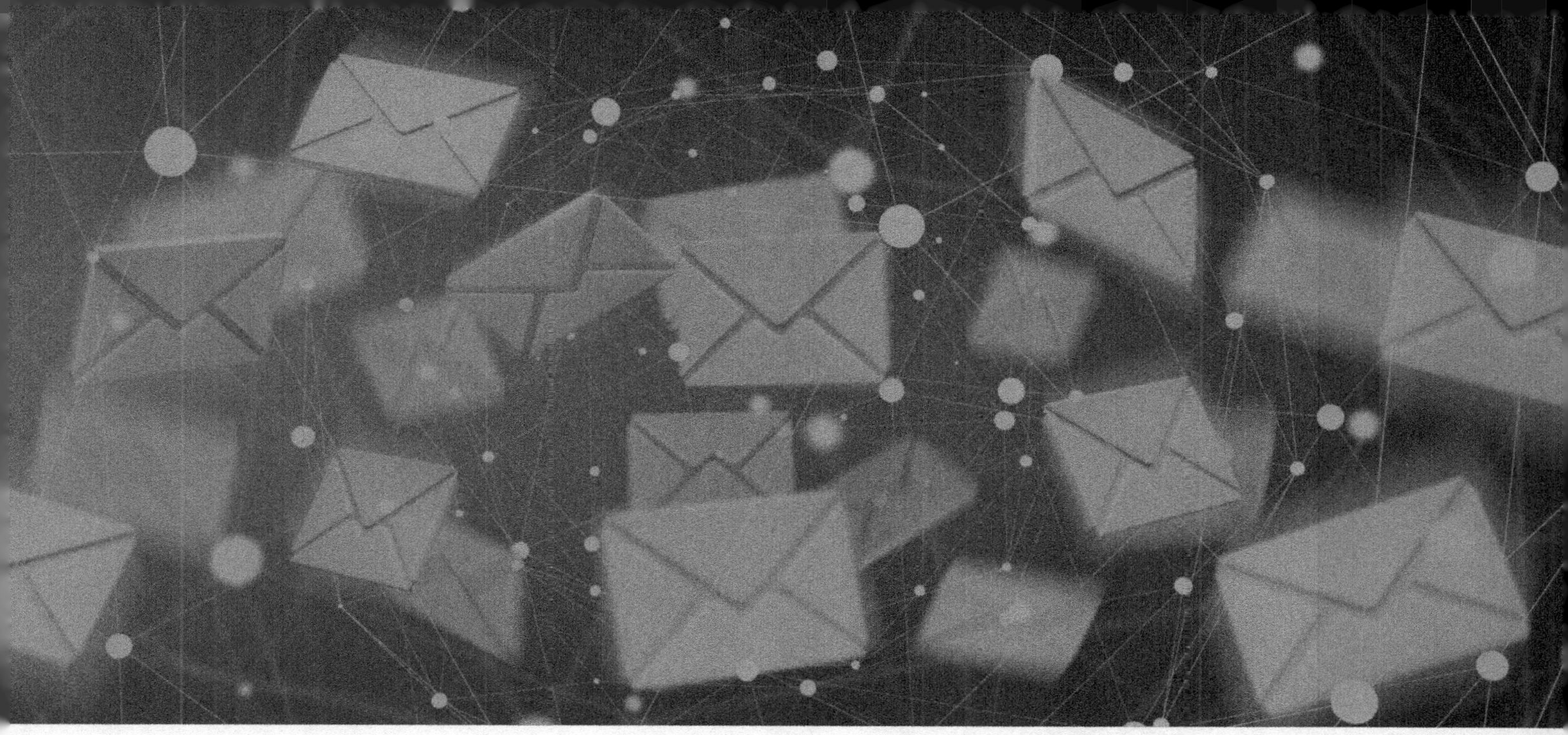

Sign up for our Newsletter

Join us @ Exam Room Tales to get a better look at what we do. We will also offer special promos and you will receive benefits for signing up for our newsletter. Our team sends out a Newsletter several times a year.

The goal of the Newsletter is to keep our readers up to date on what we are working on. It also offers a platform to provide feedback, share stories, and much more. Our Newsletter team will also offer promos, special offers, incentives, unique stories, and more.

Come Join us at ExamRoomTales.com

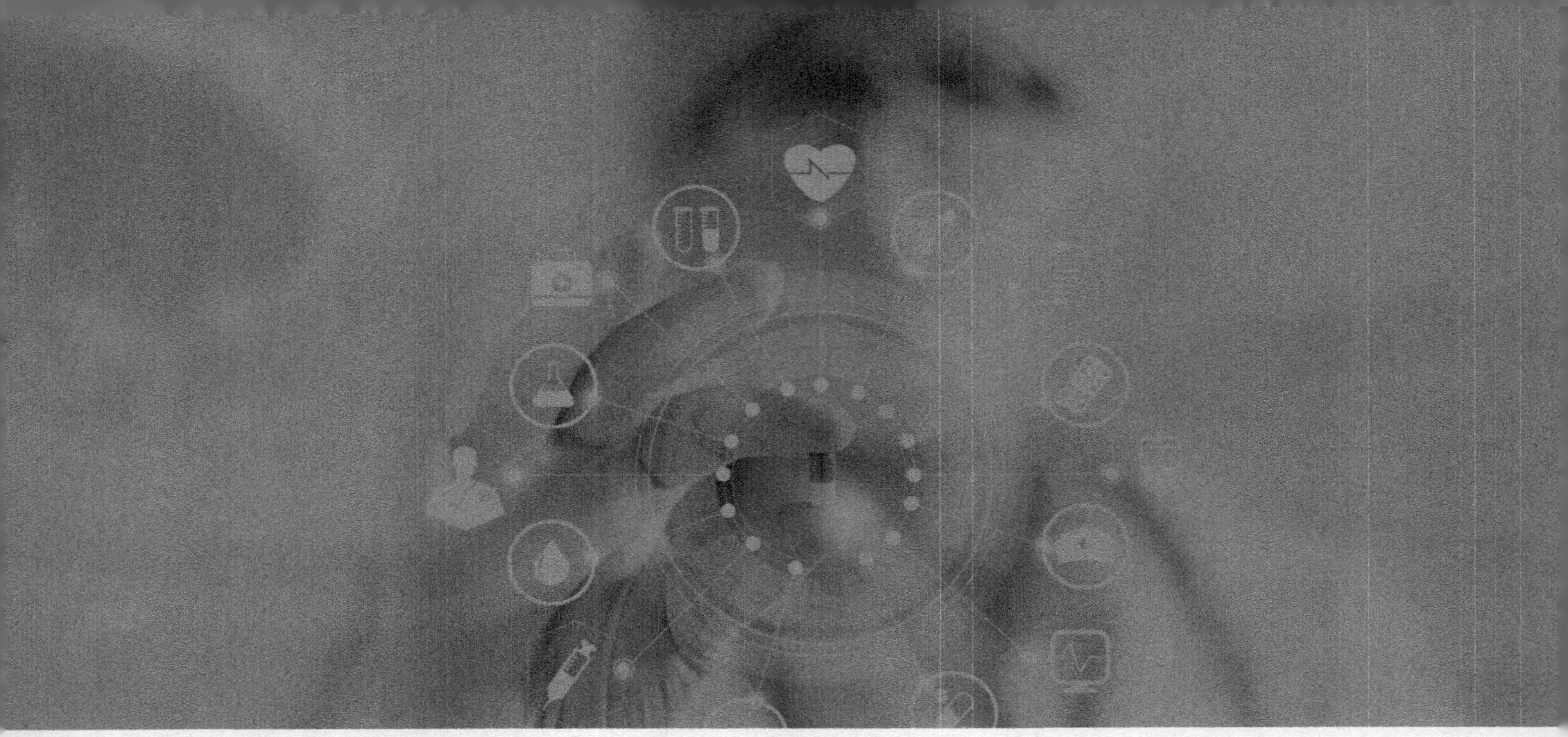

Background on Correctional Medicine in the United States

Many of our tales come from the world of prisons and jails. This is a general information sheet that we include in all our volumes. If you've read it before, please move on. However, the message is still important.

The United States has, by far, one of the highest rates of incarceration in the world. As of 2016 – 655 inmates per 100,000 are found within the jails and prisons of America. But other countries around the world are also experiencing an increase in the number of individuals incarcerated. Many different countries have tried different things to curb incarceration rates – some work, and some do not.

Each country has specific and unique ways to handle the medical needs required for inmates. This need may be overlooked or misunderstood by the general public when dealing with cost, workforce, funding, and many other areas of correctional responsibilities.

Additionally, millions of individuals have been freed from jails and prisons that are being monitored on probation or parole. This also adds to the responsibilities of the government, cities, towns, and communities. For those younger than 18 – there are often detention centers.

Correctional Medicine is challenging and unique. Inmates can be difficult to treat for several reasons, including risk factors, past medical histories, unique circumstances, unique mental health problems, difficulty following directions, homelessness, and many others. This isn't to say that every inmate falls into the category of being difficult. For some reason, the most unexpected things happen in prisons and jails.

Constitutionally, inmates should be provided with reasonable medical and mental health care. That means you can't lock them up and throw away the key. Many times, there are dental issues, pending surgeries, medications, serious medical and mental health conditions, and many more circumstances that should be considered and often continued if possible.

Not all medications that a patient takes on the streets will be allowed in a correctional facility. There are hundreds of different prisons and jails throughout the United States. This includes Federal prison/jails, state prisons, and many other forms of detention centers. Each facility will do things a little differently from one to another. This could be based on region, size, beliefs, medical knowledge, medical personnel, administration, financial, and many other things. In essence, what works for one jail may not work for another.

The medicine inside correctional facilities can be exciting, difficult, and even disturbing. It is rare when someone is satisfied with the level of care they are receiving, even if it is exceeding the standards available. Lawsuits are often brought against medical personnel, prisons, and jails. Some of these are for a good reason, but many are not.

The truth of the matter is that inmates are people and should be treated with appropriate medical care regardless of the crimes that brought them to the correctional facilities. On the opposite side of the coin, the medical staff is often attacked, berated, threatened, and more when they are trying to do the best job they can.

TALES OF THE EXAM ROOM

VOLUME - FIVE

The following stories are intended to give the reader a picture into some of the crazier and unbelievable aspects of medicine. These stories are based on true situations, but many things have been changed to protect the patient. Some stories have been combined or changed to give the reader a better understanding and picture of the world of correction medicine.

To our knowledge, all patients involved received excellent health care.

Please enjoy!!

Made in the USA
Monee, IL
08 November 2026

67948335R00050